BOBBY

THERE IS ALWAYS A LIGHT AT THE END OF THE TUNNEL

DEAR READER,

MAY YOU ALWAYS FIND THE light WHEN YOU NEED IT MOST!

REGARDS,

SSG ROBERT J. QUAYLE III (RET)

ISBN 979-8-89309-549-4 (Paperback)
ISBN 979-8-89485-422-9 (Hardcover)
ISBN 979-8-89309-550-0 (Digital)

Covenant Books
11661 Hwy 707
Murrells Inlet, SC 29576
www.covenantbooks.com

This book is dedicated to Zach, the son I never had; and to my father, the man I will never know.

Suicide Hotline numbers:

US 988

US 800-273-8255

Germany 08001810771

Belgium 02 648 40 14

Italy 800860022

Poland 5270000

Korea 080-8555-118 888-412-0470

EOD Suicide Hotline 800-931-2237

Eating Disorder Hotline 800-656-4673

National Assault Hotline 800-222-1222

Poison Control Hotline 800-799-7233 National Domestic Violence Hotline 877-565-8860

Transgender Suicide Hotline 202-498-4009

SHARP Crisis Line Text 838255 (Veterans Crisis Hotline) Text VETS to 741741 Or you can download the WeCare app for more contact and resources.

CONTENTS

Far better is it to dare mighty things, to win glorious triumphs, even though checkered by failure... than to rank with those poor spirits who neither enjoy much nor suffer much, because they live in a gray twilight that knows not victory nor defeat.

—Theodore Roosevelt

PROLOGUE

As you may know, an average of twenty-two veterans a day take their own lives. A little over ten years ago, Bobby was very nearly one of them. Bobby's life has been a tumultuous journey, filled with adversity and the constant struggle to make ends meet. Despite his many hardships, he has always managed to come out on top, and his story serves as a beacon of hope for those who may be facing similar challenges.

Growing up, Bobby faced abuse and near-death experiences, but he was always blessed with an uncanny stroke of luck that saw him through even the toughest times. After leaving high school early, he enlisted in the army and was given an amazing assignment as an intelligence analyst in Germany during the Cold War.

After serving six years in the army, Bobby embarked on a successful career in finance and banking. He opened his own financial planning firm, which eventually led to a job as a branch manager at a major bank. However, his world came crashing down twenty years later during the financial collapse of 2008, when the bank he worked for was shut down.

In a desperate bid to make ends meet, Bobby reenlisted in the army at the age of forty-three. While he was honored to serve his country once again, he suffered an injury that would ultimately lead to his medical retirement. Throughout this trying time, Bobby faced hostility and harassment from his fellow soldiers and leaders who believed that anyone who is ill or injured is automatically a "dirtbag."

Once he was medically retired, Bobby was once again left wondering what to do next. After some soul-searching, he and his wife decided to buy a retail franchise in their hometown. Running the store proved more difficult than Bobby had imagined, due to his disability, and he found himself struggling to make payroll.

One fateful day, after putting his Glock 9mm and a box of ammunition in the trunk of his car, Bobby went for a walk in the park to clear his head. He felt like a complete failure and was on the brink of taking his own life when something miraculous happened. In that moment of despair, Bobby realized that he had been given a second chance at life and that he needed to make the most of it.

Bobby's story is a testament to the human spirit and the power of perseverance. Despite facing seemingly insurmountable challenges throughout his life, he never gave up on his dreams nor lost hope for himself. His journey serves as an inspiration to anyone who may be struggling with their own hardships, and his message is clear: no matter how dreadful things may seem, there is always light at the end of the tunnel.

CHAPTER 1

You Should Write a Book

The crackle of the fire was a gentle symphony to my ears, complemented by the soothing murmur of the waterfall cascading in the background. I settled into my chair, the stone firepit's warmth enveloping me as the evening air began to carry a subtle chill. In my hand, the medical marijuana vaporizer was a lifeline, its soft hum and the faint cloud it produced standing as a testament to how far medicine—and I—had come.

As I drew a slow breath through the device, the familiar pain that laced through my body seemed to ebb, just enough for me to focus on the here and now rather than the persistent aches that told tales of a past etched with scars of service. Gone were the days when sixty milligrams of morphine would hold me hostage twice daily, leaving me adrift in a fog where time and clarity had no meaning. The vaporizer, with its dose of relief, allowed me to be present, to be more than just a shadow within my own life.

I glanced around at the life I had curated for myself, a personal sanctuary where every stone, every plant, was a choice I made, a step toward something resembling peace. The waterfall whispered secrets of resilience, each drop a memory, each ripple a challenge overcome. It was remarkable, really, how a landscape could mirror one's journey, how a backyard could become a reflection of the battles fought and the victories won.

The pain... It was my uninvited companion, a constant reminder of a fractured spine and a fractured life that I somehow managed to piece back together. Like a ghost, it followed me, but I refused to let it define me. With the vapor curling into the night air, I felt its grip loosen, granting me the space to contemplate not just the pain but the strength it took to face each day with it.

"Resilience," I murmured to myself, almost in reverence to the word. Growing up poor, facing abuse, losing everything, only to find it again in unexpected places—I carried those chapters within me, not as burdens but as proof of an indomitable spirit. My spirit. It wasn't about what life took away; it was about what I found within myself each time I was knocked down—a resolve that even I didn't know existed until the moment called for it.

As the fire danced before me, casting a warm glow on my hands, I reflected on the notion of hope. It was never about blind optimism. Hope was the stubborn, gritty belief that despite the darkness, there would be a flicker of light. And all you needed was a flicker to ignite the will to push forward, to turn the page, to start a new chapter.

"From morphine to marijuana," I whispered, a wry smile touching the corners of my mouth. "From lost to found, from despair to determination." Every puff of that vaporizer was a silent thank-you to the progress that kept me moving, to the people who stood by me when I was a mere echo of myself.

The fire crackled, reminding me that even as the wood turned to embers, it gave off the brightest light. Perhaps in sharing my story, I could be that ember for someone else—a beacon in their night, a signal that even the deepest wounds could heal, that life, like my beautifully cultivated backyard, could be reshaped into something beautiful after all.

I coaxed another deep breath from the cool evening air, letting it fill my lungs with the scent of pine and freshly turned earth. The backyard of my home is a testament to resilience—mine, nature's, the very essence of life. Surrounded by trees that stand like sentries, their branches whispering secrets to the flowers and hostas nestled at their feet, everything here is alive with a purposeful energy.

My gaze settles on the butterfly bush in the center of the yard. It is a beacon for winged creatures, hummingbirds darting through the air, their wings a blur, while butterflies flit about with an elegance that belies the turmoil they must have endured to emerge from their chrysalises. And there, near the koi pond, the dance of life continues unabated.

The pond itself, my labor of love, reflects the sky as twilight paints it in shades of orange and purple. I remember the weight of the stones in my hands, the muscle strain, the sweat—the physical echo of emotional burdens I've carried. But like this water garden, every effort was transformative.

Mickey, ever the brother in arms despite his firefighter's badge, would come over with a grin, lending not just his strength but his companionship. Mickey and his wife, Danielle, are not only great neighbors but amazing parents as well. Side by side, we created this multitiered cascade that now sings a constant melody of water meeting water.

Three large koi glide beneath the surface, their colors vibrant against the darkening waters. A largemouth bass darts out of sight, leaving ripples in its wake. The bluegill huddle together like old friends at a reunion, and I can make out the silhouettes of crayfish scuttling along the pond floor. Even the bullfrogs, those two baritones, add their voices to the night's chorus.

This is a sanctuary—not just for these creatures but for me as well. Here, amid this miniature ecosystem, I find something akin to peace. Each element of this landscape has faced its struggles—weathered storms, sought nourishment, fought for survival. Yet here they are, thriving.

"Life's a lot like gardening," I muse aloud, the vaporizer resting idle between my fingers. "You till, you plant, you nurture. Sometimes, you watch things wither… But you learn, and then you grow again."

The waterfall's steady hum is a testament to perseverance. I worked so hard to build it, stone by stone, thought by thought. Now it stands as proof that even the most ambitious projects are possible when done piece by piece, each step a small victory.

It's these victories I've gathered like the stones of my waterfall. The memories flood back, not just of pain and hardship but of the defiance against them, the refusal to remain broken. This backyard, this space filled with growth and beauty, reminds me that hope is never futile.

"From despair to determination," I repeat, letting the words hang in the warm light of the fire pit. It's true; my journey isn't one of a tranquil path but a rugged trail that has led me to vistas I could never have imagined from the valley floor.

The water falls, the fish swim, and life persists in its delicate balance. There's a majesty in that—a profound lesson in the simple act of carrying on. And as the last light of day gives way to the first star of night, I know that this is what I was meant to share. My story, like this backyard oasis, can be a refuge, a place where others might see reflections of their own resilience and find hope among the living tapestry of my words.

"Tomorrow," I resolve, "I start writing."

The fire crackled and popped, sending a cascade of sparks twirling into the evening sky. I watched as Molly and Reagan bounded across the manicured lawn, their playful yips punctuating the serene backdrop. Molly, her golden coat shimmering in the firelight, dodged left, then right, clutching the rubber tire firmly between her teeth. Reagan, sleek and agile, feinted with precision, her dark eyes locked onto the prize. They were an embodiment of relentless joy, two spirits unburdened by the weight of the past, living fully in the chase.

I leaned back in my chair, a plume of scented vapor rising from my lips as I exhaled slowly. Medical marijuana—a far cry from the morphine haze that once clouded my existence—offered clarity and a respite from the pain. It allowed moments like these to be more than just a fleeting distraction; they were a chance to reflect, to appreciate.

"You should write a book," the echo of countless passengers reverberated in my mind, their words tumbling through my thoughts as though they were seated beside me now. My time behind the wheel of the Cadillac CT6 had been more than just a job; it was a stage for my life's tales, a confessional where strangers became momentary confidants. And each time I shared a piece of my journey, there was a spark of something undefinable—an exchange of humanity that lingered long after the ride ended.

"Maybe they're right," I mused, watching the dogs' relentless game. Their tenacity mirrored my own determination, the same spirit that saw me through darkness and into light. Their refusal to let go of the tire they were playing with felt symbolic, a reminder that I, too, had held on when everything seemed intent on pulling me under.

"Stories," I whispered, "everyone has them." But mine were etched with the kind of truth that comes from having danced with despair and come out leading the waltz. Could my stories, woven into the fabric of a book, serve as a beacon for others? Was it possible that the lessons I've learned could guide someone else through their night?

A gentle breeze carried the scent of pine and blooming flowers, mingling with the earthy aroma of the fire. It was a fragrance of growth, of life persisting despite the odds. Yes, my backyard paradise bore witness to my labor, but it was also a testament to the power of nurturing hope.

"Tomorrow," I affirmed as the dogs finally collapsed into a panting heap, the tire abandoned momentarily in their exhaustion, "I'll start putting pen to paper."

In this stillness, with the symphony of nature playing softly around me, I knew that the stories I carried—the laughter, the tears, the triumphs, and the scars—were not just mine to hold. They were a gift, a roadmap of resilience meant to be shared. And if hope could bloom here, in this little corner of the world, then surely it could take root in the pages I was yet to write.

The crackle of the fire seemed to synchronize with the slow, methodical tapping of my foot against the stone patio—a metronome to my thoughts. Molly and Reagan had succumbed to their exhaustion, lying side by side, their chests heaving in the afterglow of play. I took another draw from the vaporizer, letting the calm wash over me.

It was in moments like this, surrounded by the tranquil beauty I had cultivated, that my past unfurled before me—my own private panorama of struggles and victories.

I'd been an intelligence analyst for the army, not once but twice. The first stint carved out the early years of my adult life; the second, a desperate pivot when the world's economy faltered, and the bank doors shuttered for good. At forty-three, the mirror reflected someone who had traded military discipline for corporate comfort. Fifty pounds had to melt away—each one shed through gritted teeth and pounding heartbeats—as I prepared to don the uniform again. It wasn't just about getting back into shape; it was a reclaiming of identity, a rekindling of purpose.

As my gaze settled on the dancing flames, I could almost feel the heat of the Afghan sun, a deployment that never came to pass. Instead, my battle turned inward when a training accident shattered not just my spine but the future I had envisioned in service to my country. The sterile smell of the hospital, the antiseptic sting of despair—I had breathed it all as surgeons worked to piece me back together.

Recovery was a word too sterile for the grueling journey back to mobility. Learning to walk again was a testament to human willpower—every step a silent declaration of war against my own limitations. But some battles leave you forever changed. And so, medically retired, I returned to civilian life with a spine held together more by sheer determination than by bone.

The soft glow of the embers now reflected off the pond's still surface, and I thought of how my life mirrored these waters. Beneath the tranquility, there had always been movement, life teeming in the depths—koi turning lazy circles, the occasional ripple as a bullfrog leapt to safety. Resilience isn't just surviving; it's thriving in spite of what seeks to pull you under.

A whisper of wind rustled through the pines, as if urging me on. Yes, I would share these stories. My time in the army, the years threading through the fabric of finance, and the reawakening of the soldier within when duty called again. These weren't just recollections; they were beacons for those navigating their own darkness.

"Tomorrow," I murmured, the promise a pact with myself. With each word I would write, I'd offer up pieces of my soul—not for accolades or acclaim but for the chance that someone, somewhere, might see their reflection in my trials and recognize the spark of their own undying hope.

The scent of pine, the sound of the waterfall, the warmth of the fire—they were all reminders of life's relentless march. And just like the koi in the pond, no matter how confined we feel by our circumstances, we can—and must—keep moving through the water, under the open sky of possibility.

The fire crackled, a companion to my thoughts as I settled deeper into the Adirondack chair, its wooden arms worn smooth by seasons of reflection. Wisps of smoke curled upward, dissipating into the evening sky, carrying with them the tales of two decades spent amid ledgers and loans. At twenty-three, my hands had already been stained with ink, signing off on dreams, on homes, on futures—a young president of a financial planning firm, an even younger leader at the chamber of commerce.

"Who would believe it?" I chuckled softly, the sound lost in the symphony of Molly and Reagan's playful barks. "A kid from nowhere, balancing books and shaking hands with the city's stalwarts."

The vaporizer, light between my fingers, was a lifeline back from the depths of pain and memory. The medicinal haze was less about forgetting and more about grounding, about sifting through the sediment of life for the gold flecks of wisdom hard-earned.

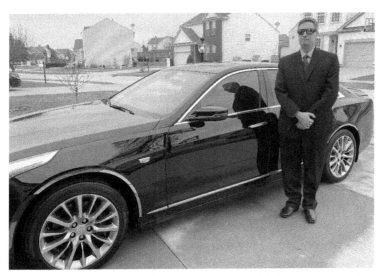

This is me getting ready to drive my new black Cadillac CT6 for Uber Black, their premium service in the Cleveland area. My passengers provided the encouragement that I needed to write this book.

"Write a book, Bobby," echoed the voices of strangers, faces blurred in the rearview mirror of my Cadillac, their stories as transient as their presence in my journey. Each one saw a spark in the mundane, a reason to chronicle the highs and inevitable lows. But self-doubt is a shroud that dims even the brightest of sparks.

"Why should I write a book? Nobody cares," I whispered to the night, the words a mix of question and indictment. My gaze drifted to the butterfly bush—its blooms a riot of color, a testament to beauty born from the dirt. I thought of the countless others out there, wrestling with their own doubts, their stories untold, unseen. Could mine serve as a beacon? A lighthouse guiding weary travelers through the fog of uncertainty?

"Maybe they do care," I conceded, the realization dawning like the first light of morning across a troubled sea. "Maybe it's not about the grandeur of the tale but the truth in the telling."

I rose, brushing off the remnants of hesitation. The fire needed tending, much like the narrative weaving through my mind. Each log placed upon the flames was symbolic—an act of building, of nurturing potential. I watched the sparks fly upward, each one a fleeting chance, a possibility, an idea that could ignite a soul against the dark.

"Tomorrow," I affirmed, the word a silent vow cast into the future. I would begin to write—not for fortune, not for fame, but for the solitary soul searching for a sign that someone else has weathered the storm and emerged, not unscathed, but undefeated.

The embers glowed, a heart beating beneath the ashes, and I knew that resilience isn't merely surviving—it's sharing your survival, so others might live too.

The crackling of the fire was a soothing symphony to my ears, punctuated by the occasional splash from the water garden. I pulled in a deep breath, the cool night air mingling with the scent of pine and smoldering wood. My mind began to drift, unanchored from the present comfort of my backyard, sailing back through the murky waters of memory to a day that had nearly been my last.

I could almost feel the damp earth beneath me as I sat there, swallowed by the shadows of the Metroparks. The leaves whispered secrets to one another, oblivious to the despair that clung to me like a second skin. There, surrounded by the indifferent beauty of nature, I cradled failure in my hands—the retail business I had bet everything on was crumbling before my eyes, and so was my marriage. I had been proud, confident, but reality tore through those illusions, leaving me raw and exposed.

The cold metal of the gun pressed against my temple was a stark contrast to the softness of the forest floor. My finger rested on the trigger, heavy with intention. It would have been so easy to just give in, to let the silence take me. But then, piercing the stillness, what I would define as a miracle occurred. A song filled the woods around me—a melody so clear and poignant it felt like an intervention.

Was it a sign? A coincidence? It didn't matter. In that moment, a plea for divine intervention became my lifeline. The song tethered me back to reality, pulling me away from the precipice upon which I teetered.

I lowered the gun, my hand trembling, not with fear but with the sudden rush of hope. The music continued, wrapping around me like a warm embrace, and I made the decision to rise. To walk out of those woods. To go home.

Now, as I tended to the fire, placing another log onto the glowing embers, I reflected on the incredible journey that had brought me here. The stone pit, with its dancing flames, was like an altar to my past trials—a place where I could lay down my burdens and watch them transform into something else, something useful—warmth, light, insight.

"Maybe it's not about the grandeur of the tale but the truth in the telling," I murmured into the night. That song, that intervention, was a testament to the unseen forces that guide us, the threads of connection that bind us all. It was a reminder that life can turn on the smallest of moments and that sometimes help comes in the most unexpected forms.

With a newfound resolve, I stood up, my gaze fixed on the stars peeking through the canopy of pines. I would write my book, not as a monument to myself but as a beacon for others lost in their own dark woods. If my story could be the song that reached someone when they needed it most, then every word would be worth writing.

"Tomorrow," I whispered to the silent guardians of my solace. The dogs, sensing a shift in my mood, settled down near my feet, their presence a comforting weight. *Tomorrow, I will begin.* And perhaps, in the sharing of my darkest hour, I could offer a sliver of light to those still searching for their way home.

The fire crackled and popped, sending a shower of sparks skyward as I poked at the embers with an old iron rod. The warmth on my face was a stark contrast to the cool dampness settling around me. My eyes were wet, not from the smoke but from memories that cascaded through my mind like the waterfall behind me. "God bless her," I whispered into the evening air, the name Carrie Underwood a solemn prayer on my lips.

As the scent of burning pine mingled with the earthy aroma of the surrounding grasses, my heart throbbed against my rib cage, each beat a reminder of the life I almost threw away. That day in the Metroparks was etched into my brain, the cold steel of the gun a chilling memory against the temple of a man who had lost all hope. My finger, which once trembled on the trigger, now shook for a different reason—for the overwhelming flood of gratitude and the realization of what might have been lost.

Her voice had pierced the suffocating silence of despair, a lifeline thrown across the abyss. It was more than just a song—it was a sign, a moment of divine intervention when I needed it most.

I leaned back in my chair, watching Molly and Reagan chase each other in playful circles, their joyful barking a stark juxtaposition to the somber reflection gripping me. They were oblivious to the weight of human sorrow, living entirely in the moment, and I envied them for it. But even as I watched them, an epiphany dawned on me as bright and startling as the flames before me.

That's why I need to write the book! The thought came unbidden, surging forth with the force of a revelation. A book could be my melody, my lyrics to reach out through the darkness. If my life's tumultuous symphony could resonate with just one person teetering on the brink, then every hardship I endured would gain a new purpose.

The possibility felt like a second chance—not only for me but for anyone who might read my story. What if my words could be the thread pulling someone back from the edge? What if they could inspire resilience where there was resignation or kindle hope in a place grown cold with despair?

It wouldn't be about crafting a bestseller or earning accolades; this would be a chronicle of survival, a testament to the power of perseverance. I wanted to show that no pit was too deep, no night too dark that couldn't be overcome. And maybe, just maybe, my tale could serve as proof that things do get better, often far beyond what we might imagine.

"Tomorrow," I said again, a vow cast into the night—a promise to myself and to any unseen forces listening. With each word I would pen, I intended to build a bridge across the chasms of hopelessness, a pathway back to the light.

As the last glimmer of daylight surrendered to the evening stars, I knew that my journey wasn't just mine anymore. It belonged to every struggling soul searching for a sign. And so with the gentle hum of nature as my witness, I embraced the destiny that beckoned: to share my story, to offer up my pain and triumphs, in the hopes of lighting the way for others. Tomorrow, the work will begin.

The crackling fire before me seemed to dance in agreement with my racing thoughts. Flames licked the sky as if reaching toward the stars that had been silent witnesses to my life's trials and tribulations. I leaned back in my chair, the heat warming my face—a stark contrast to the chills of memories that ran down my spine.

Growing up, my world was a canvas of grays—no silver linings—just a boy without a father, a home marred by absence and silent cries. Poverty wasn't just a word; it was the fabric of my clothes, the emptiness of our fridge, the hollow echo in my mother's sighs. The abuse, a shadow that followed me long after I stepped into the light, taught me to flinch before I learned to reach out for comfort.

They say what doesn't kill you makes you stronger, but they don't tell you how much it can hurt, how scars can itch years after they've healed. Divorce papers stacked like layers of fallen leaves, twice over, each one a season of love lost, and trust betrayed. Bankruptcy—not once but twice—the bitter taste of failure that no amount of rinsing could cleanse.

And then there was the army, my crucible, where I found camaraderie and conflict in equal measure. Hostility wasn't just from the enemy lines; it came from within, questioning my worth after the accident. The day my spine fractured was the day my spirit was put to the test, forging a resilience I never knew I possessed. Learning to walk again wasn't just about putting one foot in front of the other—it was about standing tall when every fiber of your being wants to stay down.

But through all this, there was something that anchored me. I think back to those movies, the ones with Rocky Balboa, a fighter not because he chose to be but because life gave him no other option. Those words he said, they were more than just lines—they were the mantra of my existence, the battle cry that echoed in the silence of my darkest nights.

Rocky Balboa—every underdog's champion. His voice resonated within me now, rousing memories of a younger Bobby, sitting cross-legged on a worn-out carpet, eyes wide and heart pounding as he watched the Italian Stallion rise and fall and rise again.

"The world ain't all sunshine and rainbows," Rocky said, his image flickering on the old television set that was our window to worlds beyond our cramped apartment. I could almost feel the gruffness of his voice, a counterpoint to the symphonic sounds of the waterfall behind me. "It's a very mean and nasty place."

"Life's tough," I whispered to myself, feeling the weight of my past and the promise of my future simultaneously heavy and uplifting on my shoulders. "But so am I."

It seems almost foolish now, the idea of encapsulating such a tumultuous life within the confines of mere pages. How do you compress decades of pain, hope, loss, and triumph into chapters and sentences? How do you translate tears and laughter, despair, and joy into words that strangers might read and find solace in?

Maybe it's not about the quantity, I mused, watching a lone ember escape the pit and float upward, joining the stars. *Maybe it's about the honesty of each word, the raw truth behind each story.*

My hands found warmth in the glow of the fire, and I realized that warmth could spread beyond this backyard sanctuary. I could offer it to others, those shivering in the cold of their own life's winters, searching for a spark to reignite their hope.

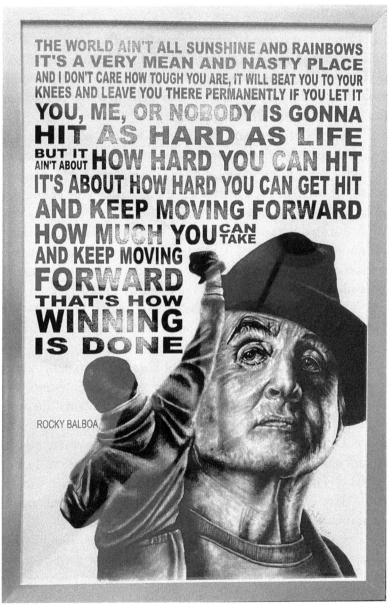

This artwork was given to me by the artist, Cyril Kleem who is the mayor of the fine city of Berea, OH, where much of my story takes place.

The night wrapped around me like a blanket as I visualized the path ahead—not paved but a trail blazed by sheer will. Each step forward would be a word, each chapter a milestone. My story would be a beacon, its purpose far greater than self-reflection.

Tomorrow, I thought, the whisper of the waterfall mingling with the rustle of the pines. *Tomorrow, I begin the journey anew—not just for me, but for anyone who needs to hear that yes, things can get better. Much better than you ever imagined.*

"Life's about how hard you can get hit and keep moving forward," echoed Rocky's voice in my head. That quote had become a mantra for me, a north star guiding me through the darkest nights of my soul. It brought back memories of every fall, every failure that I had faced down and overcome.

As I stirred the embers of the fire, a figure approached—the soft steps familiar and welcome. Cheryl, my wife, her face illuminated by the flickering light, sat beside me. A smile touched my lips as our eyes met, a silent acknowledgment of the bond we shared.

"What are you thinking about?" she asked, her voice gentle against the symphony of nature around us. She noticed the moisture in my eyes, concern etched on her features.

"Just thinking about all the stuff I have been through," I began, my gaze returning to the fire. "And if writing a book about it would help anyone or not." My voice trailed off as I considered the weight of my words, the lives that might find direction from my journey. "It's something I have been kicking around for a few years now, and I just can't shake the feeling that it is something that I MUST do."

Cheryl nodded, her hand finding mine, an anchor in the sea of doubt. "Honey, do you think it's because it will stop someone from killing themselves?"

The starkness of her words hung between us, mingling with the smoke that rose steadily into the night. I knew she understood, perhaps better than anyone, the gravity of what I was contemplating. The thought of reaching out from the pages of a yet-unwritten book, to grip the hand of someone teetering on the edge of despair, felt like a responsibility I couldn't ignore.

"Maybe that's it," I said finally, a resolve settling within me. "If my story could lead just one person back from that brink, then every word I write...every memory I relive...it'll be worth it."

The fire popped and hissed, as if in agreement, and I watched the sparks ascend toward the heavens, tiny beacons of light against the overwhelming dark. *Tomorrow, I will begin. Not just for myself but for those still searching for a flicker of hope in their own darkness. Tomorrow, I will take another hit and keep moving forward because that's how winning is done.*

Cradling the warmth of the fire in my palms, I watched the flames dance with a life of their own. Cheryl sat down beside me, her presence a reassuring weight against my side. Six years had passed since we exchanged vows, yet every day with her felt like a reaffirmation of something sacred, something that had once seemed as elusive as the smoke curling skyward.

"Cheryl, you've seen me at my worst," I began, the words tumbling out with an urgency born of countless nights wrestling with doubt. "You were there when the world seemed to have run out of second chances for me."

She squeezed my hand, a silent gesture that spoke volumes of the support she'd never withheld, not even when our life together was punctuated by the echoes of my past traumas. "Bobby, you're one of the strongest people I know. Authoring this book...it's not just about healing yourself. It's also about offering a lifeline to others who are drowning in despair."

I nodded, the idea settling into the spaces between my ribs, wrapping around my heart. *Therapeutic* was the word she used, and it resonated within me—a promise of redemption through the act of sharing my story.

"Making money from the book isn't the goal," I said, watching the fireflies begin their nightly ballet among the darkening trees. "If my words can stop even one person from feeling so alone that they think ending their life is the only answer, then I'll have succeeded beyond any measure of wealth or fame."

A gentle smile touched her lips, softening her features in the glow of the embers. Cheryl worked tirelessly, juggling her job and the care of her two daughters, ensuring they received the education and opportunities she fought so hard for. Her dedication was another kind of fire, one that fueled our hopes for a future where we could both lay down our burdens.

"Once the girls are on their feet, self-sufficient, and strong just like their mother, we'll have time," she murmured, gazing into the flames. "We'll retire, and maybe then your book will be out there, changing lives."

Her words were a balm soothing the raw edges of my ambition. We didn't need grandeur or accolades. We had each other, and that was enough. And perhaps in the quiet aftermath of our working years, we would find solace in knowing that our struggles—the hits we took and kept moving forward from—might guide someone else through their darkest hour.

"Winning is done one step at a time," I whispered to myself, my eyes tracing the flight of a lone moth as it circled closer to the light. Tomorrow, I would take another step by starting my book, driven by hope, buoyed by love, and eternally grateful for the sheer luck of being alive to tell the tale.

CHAPTER 2

A NEW BEGINNING

The gentle warmth from the gas fireplace in the corner of my living room countered the chill from the window, while the low hum of a nature documentary played on my eighty-five-inch ultra-HD television. My laptop sat before me, the cursor blinking patiently on a blank document as I poised my fingers over the keys. After hours of rambunctious play, my faithful dogs had settled into a serene quietude beside me, only occasionally stirring to nudge my hand for attention or a treat.

Retirement wraps around me like a well-worn blanket—comfortable and secure. With no pressing schedule, I have the luxury of time, an abundance that I channel into the book that's been simmering in my mind. The attempt at resuming a career in banking was brief, the familiar walls of the institution closing in on me faster than I could have anticipated. Stress, like an unwelcome shadow, loomed over tasks I once performed with ease. Yet it wasn't just the tediousness of spreadsheets and interest rates that drove me away. There was a pulsating need to do something more meaningful—this book.

Sitting here, the soft click-clack of the keyboard under my fingertips, I'm reminded of the freedom that my military pension and benefits afford me. They're not just monetary security, they are a gateway to pursue this dream without the constraints of necessity. I didn't need to stand behind a counter again; I needed to tell my story. A tale not of a man defined by his past but one who continuously forges ahead.

The dogs, sensing my contemplative mood, lay their heads back down, their breathing synchronized with the flickering flames. It's in this tranquility that I find the courage to dive into the "meat and potatoes" of my journey. The beginning, when I was a child, feels like both a distant memory and a vivid scar.

"Let's begin," I murmur to the empty room, my voice intermingling with the crackle of the fire. And so with a deep breath, I start to type, hopeful that my experiences might, one day, light the path for others walking through their own darkness. This isn't just a recollection of what was; it is a beacon for what can be—a manuscript of resilience, hope, and perhaps even a bit of luck and divine intervention.

The soft light from my laptop screen casts a glow on my hands as they glide over the keyboard, each keystroke adding to the peaceful melody of my living room. I lean back in my chair and release a satisfied sigh. My eyes wander toward the cards scattered on the browser tab, an online recreation of the poker table where I've honed my skills for hours on end. As I work on the beginning of my unfinished story, I continue to play Texas Hold'em passively in the background.

Texas Hold'em Poker isn't just a pastime; it's a discipline. Over a dozen books with creased spines sit on my shelf, their pages dog-eared from frequent consultation. The master classes I took online didn't just teach me about odds and outs; they illuminated the intricate ballet of risk and reward. And through it all, my coach—whose voice crackles through the speakers during our sessions—has been a steadfast mentor, guiding me closer to my ambition.

"Patience, Bobby," I remind myself, my thoughts drifting to the televised tournament that has long since been etched into my bucket list. The entry fee—a steep mountain of cash—is beyond my reach, but I've always believed in earning my place at the table. Nearly a decade's worth of practice is narrowing the gap between dream and reality. It's not if but when I'll claim that seat and look into the camera with a steady gaze, my hand steady as I lay down my cards.

Rising from my chair, I stretch my legs and wander to my basement sanctuary. There, nestled amid the mechanical hum of filters and the gentle burble of water, is my 125-gallon freshwater aquarium. A world within glass walls, it thrives quietly, mirroring the balance I seek in life and poker. Cichlids glide through their aquatic terrain, each movement deliberate and serene. They know nothing of the stakes outside their submerged Eden nor do they need to. Their simplicity is a lesson in itself.

In the dim light, I pull up a stool and cradle a warm mug between my palms, the aroma of coffee mingling with the earthy scent of aquatic plants. This is where I come to reflect, to strategize, and sometimes to simply be. Each bubble that rises to the surface is a reminder that even in stillness, there is progress, a subtle push toward what lies ahead.

There are days when the weight of unfulfilled aspirations threatens to anchor me down, but in this tranquil space, hope finds its way back, buoyant and resilient. For every setback, there is a step forward, for every loss a lesson learned. And as the daylight fades, giving way to the hushed tones of evening, I find solace in the knowledge that every hand played, every decision made, is another ripple in the pond of my existence, moving me ever closer to the shores of success.

The gentle hum of the aquarium's filter melds with the rhythmic ticking of the wall clock, grounding me in the present as I contemplate the past. My fingertips graze the cool glass, tracing the slow dance of the cichlids as they weave through their underwater forest. Each stroke is a silent acknowledgment of the journey that led me here, to this moment of introspection.

Over a decade has passed since my career in the military ended—not with a flourish but with the muted tones of necessity. The realization that my body could no longer keep pace with my ambitions was a bitter pill, one that forced me to reimagine my path. It was then, harnessing what remained of my resolve, that I sought refuge in education, leveraging the GI Bill into a shield against stagnation.

I remember the pride that swelled in my chest when my name was called, not once but twice, as I walked across those academic stages. *Magna cum laude*—words that echoed achievements and hinted at promise, even as my body protested each step. Intelligence operations—a field ripe with intrigue, now an untrodden path shadowed by the reality of my physical limitations.

"Adapt and overcome," I murmur, the mantra slipping from my lips as it has countless times before. It's a phrase that has threaded itself through the fabric of my life, a constant companion whispering resilience in the face of adversity.

Now a new challenge beckons: the blank pages of my book, a canvas awaiting the first strokes of my story. The cursor blinks expectantly on the laptop screen, a metronome keeping time with my thoughts. Where does one begin when every memory clamors for attention, each demanding its place in the narrative tapestry?

With a sigh, I lean back and let my gaze settle on the tranquil scene before me. The fish glide effortlessly, unburdened by doubt or fear, each movement a testament to the power of instinct and adaptation. Perhaps that's where the answer lies—in the simplicity of being, in the courage to move forward despite the murky waters ahead.

And so the decision settles within me, clear and unforced. I'll start at the very beginning, drawing from the well of childhood memories. There, nestled between innocence and experience, lie the seeds of who I would become—a man defined not by his disabilities but by the sheer force of will to rise above them.

"From small beginnings come great things," I whisper to the room, the weight of the words buoying my spirit. With renewed determination, I turn to the keyboard, fingers poised to unlock the past, to share the tale of a boy who faced the world head-on and emerged, if not unscathed, then certainly unbowed.

"Let's begin," I say as much to myself as to the quiet listeners beneath the water's surface. And with a click, the journey unfolds.

CHAPTER 3

A TROUBLED CHILDHOOD

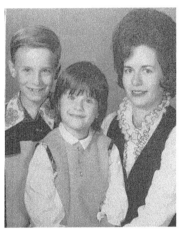

My mother Elaine, sister Deborah, and me.

I remember the sharpness of the gravel beneath my sneakers, each step a reluctant march closer to that place I called home. My heart would pound against my ribs, a frantic drumbeat echoing the terror that gripped me. With every footfall, my small frame trembled, and by the time our dilapidated porch came into view, a familiar warmth spread down my legs, the fabric clinging coldly to my skin.

The shame of it was heavy, a wet reminder of the fear that soaked into my very being. Yet in those moments, I found a strange solace in the predictable rhythm of dread and release. It became a ritual—school, walk, fear, wet pants—a cycle I had no power to break.

"Almost there, Bobby," I'd whisper to myself, summoning the courage to face what lay beyond our creaky front door. The sight of the house made my stomach churn, but somewhere deep inside, a spark of stubborn hope flickered.

My mother, Elaine, never knew the full extent of the horrors that awaited me when the school bell rang its daily goodbye. She was battling her own demons, trying to stitch together a life for us with threadbare resources and frayed determination. But even she couldn't miss the telltale signs of a child living in silent agony.

When she finally noticed the pattern—my soiled clothes, my jittery demeanor—her eyes filled with a pain so profound it seemed to crack the foundation of her world. She held me close that day, her arms a fortress around my shivering body, and whispered promises of change.

"Nothing is going to hurt you anymore, Bobby. I won't let it," she insisted with a conviction that cut through my despair like a beacon.

I clung to her words, a lifeline thrown across the chasm of my experiences, daring to believe that maybe, just maybe, the future could be different. That belief became the bedrock upon which I built my resilience.

And now, decades later, as I recount these fragmented memories to a blank page meant to inspire others, I realize how that resilience has defined me. How it taught me to walk through storms with my head held high, knowing that clear skies must eventually follow. How it gave me the strength to keep moving forward, one faltering step at a time, toward a life crafted by my own hands.

"Hope is a powerful thing," I scribble down, my pen racing across the paper, making notes for the story now unfolding on the screen before me. "It's the belief in a tomorrow that holds more promise than the yesterdays we've survived. It's the understanding that while we can't choose where we come from, we can choose where we go."

I pause, taking a deep breath as I feel the weight of my past lighten. The boy who once trudged home in fear has journeyed far, and though the path was riddled with pitfalls and shadows, he has emerged into the light of his own making.

"Keep pushing forward," I write, my heart swelling with the truth of those words. "Because sometimes, luck isn't just about chance. It's about fighting until the odds start to favor you."

With that, I set the laptop down, lean back in my chair, and allow myself a moment to simply be. To appreciate the quiet triumph of a spirit unbroken by the monsters of its past. A testament to the enduring power of hope, resilience, and, yes, a little bit of luck.

*****

I remember the day the letter came. The San Antonio sun was unforgiving, a harsh glare against the windowpanes as I sat playing with my toy soldiers on the linoleum floor, blissfully unaware of the seismic shift about to occur. My mother's hands trembled as she unfolded the paper, a foreign script dancing across its surface—that much I could tell even at that tender young age. Her face, usually so composed, crumbled like an ancient cliff worn down by relentless tides.

"Everything all right, Mama?" I asked, looking up from my imaginary battlefield. She attempted a smile, but it didn't reach her eyes, and she quickly ushered me back to my play without an answer.

My father had been a distant figure, more a myth than a man, his uniform hanging in the closet long after he'd stopped filling it. When the reality of his transgressions arrived in our mailbox—an ocean away but cutting deep—my mother made a choice that would brand us outcasts in our own community.

In those days, divorce wasn't just a family matter; it was a scandal. Our small church, once a sanctuary, became a court of judgment. I clutched my sister's hand as we walked through the doors, feeling the weight of stares, the whispers snaking around us like vipers. *Bastard* was not a word I fully understood then, but I felt its sting, delivered from the pastor's lips with righteous venom that confused and terrified me.

"God loves all his children," my mother whispered to us, defiant though her voice quivered. She held her head high, her spine straight as the oak outside our window, even as we were escorted from the pews where we once sang hymns and read scripture. I couldn't comprehend it then, the cruelty of being shunned for sins not our own, but it planted a seed within me—a determination to prove them wrong.

Alone but for each other, my mother, sister, and I forged a new path. Through whispered slurs and sideways glances, we walked on. And in the quiet moments, when the dusk painted the sky in shades of hope, my mother would hold me close and speak of brighter days ahead.

"Life isn't fair, Bobby," she'd say, her fingers combing through my hair. "But that doesn't mean we can't be brave. We make our luck by never giving up by facing each day with courage and love."

That resilience has carried me, shaping the man I've grown into. As I reflect on our journey, writing these memories onto the page, I realize that our trials, while heavy, have also been our greatest teachers. Each challenge faced, each barrier overcome, has been a testament to the power of hope.

"Mother was right," I muse aloud, the echo of her wisdom still fresh. "We are the architects of our fate, building from the rubble, crafting something beautiful from the broken."

Sunlight filters through the blinds of my living room, casting lines of gold across my laptop. In their warmth, I find a peace hard-won, a quiet triumph over the shadows of the past. The world may have labeled us outcasts, but we wore it as armor, and it has made all the difference.

I sit at the worn kitchen table, the hum of the refrigerator a steady backdrop to my thoughts as I turn the pages of our family album—a visual saga of struggle and triumph. The photos are faded now, much like the memories they encapsulate. But their message remains clear, imprinted in my very soul: never give up.

In one such photograph, my mother stands in front of our old apartment building, her eyes determined, lips set in a firm line. She's clutching a briefcase, her armor against a world that told her she didn't belong in the workforce. We were very poor back then, not because of laziness or lack of ambition but because women weren't paid well. It was an era when society expected them to be barefoot and pregnant at home, not out working jobs meant for men. Yet there she stood, defying every stereotype, the epitome of resilience.

Each day, she rose before dawn, her routine a silent protest against the injustices of the time. I remember the sound of the coffee pot gurgling as she prepared for battle, her silhouette framed by the dim kitchen light. My sister and I would pretend to sleep, listening to the soft rustle of papers as she reviewed her grievance against the US Government. A fight for equal pay—a fight that seemed endless.

"Life is often a marathon, not a sprint," she'd remind us whenever we saw her spirit wane. Her resolve was like something out of a movie, akin to Rocky Balboa's relentless pursuit of victory. And eventually, after years of tireless effort and a room full of paperwork, she won. But it was a bittersweet victory; no damages, just the promotion she had earned without any back pay. How could this be fair? An underdog's win, yet the system still held the upper hand.

We lived in a modest reality, our circumstances threadbare but our dignity intact. Times when the cupboards grew empty, Mother would somehow conjure a meal, her ingenuity nothing short of magic. "We may not have much," she'd say, "but we have each other, and that's more than enough." And it was. Through her actions, she taught us that wealth wasn't counted in coins but in character.

As I close the album, I lean back in my chair, allowing the weight of the past to settle. My mother's journey was fraught with loneliness, especially after my sister and I ventured out on our own. She never did remarry, choosing instead a solitary existence—a warrior queen without her court. Yet even in solitude, she exuded strength, a beacon guiding us through life's tumultuous seas.

My hand hovers over the laptop, ready to transpose these reflections into words that might inspire others. Our story isn't unique, but it speaks to the indomitable human spirit that persists against all odds. Our lives, rough-hewn by adversity, stand as evidence that hope can flourish in the most barren of soils.

"From hardship, we glean the seeds of our future," I write on my notepad, my handwriting a mirror of my mother's—steady and sure. I pause, allowing myself a small smile. Yes, we were dirt poor, but in the richest sense, we were millionaires of the heart. In the end, isn't that the true measure of prosperity?

The sun dips lower, casting a golden hue across the room. Shadows dance along the walls, retreating as the light asserts itself—a daily reminder that darkness is transient, and brightness always returns. It is in this ebb and flow that I find a metaphor for our lives, a testament to the enduring power of hope.

"Mother," I whisper, though she isn't here to hear me, "you were right. We make our luck, one unwavering step at a time."

The papers fluttered like fallen leaves on the kitchen table, a tumultuous history laid bare. There they were—the legal documents from her long fight with the government, the court rulings, and the letters of retaliation, each one a scar etched into our family's narrative, yet she had faced them all with the ferocity of a lioness protecting her cubs.

"Life," she would say, "isn't about waiting for the storm to pass. It's learning to dance in the rain." And dance she did, through every thunderclap of injustice and each flash flood of adversity. When the government pushed back, trying to wear down her spirit with their bureaucratic weight, she didn't flinch or falter. She took them to court. And even though the victory was more moral than material, it was enough to make them back off.

Retirement came not as a retreat but as a strategic withdrawal. My mother's resilience wasn't about pride; it was survival, an act of preserving her dignity against the relentless grind of time and toil. At eighty-two, her body is now a map of battles fought and won—every wrinkle a trench, every age spot a medal of honor.

When the heart attack seized her, the paramedics had to wrestle death away as it coiled around her, greedy for another soul. But she returned, her pulse a steady drumbeat defiant of the Reaper's rhythm. Then COVID-19 tried to claim her in the sterile battlefield of the hospital, where the air itself was thick with invisible enemies. She emerged again, victorious but weary. And when the stroke threatened to steal her voice and movement, she fought with the silence of her mind until words and steps returned to her command.

Knocked down thrice, stood up four times, I muse, tracing the veins on my own hands, a genetic testament to her indomitable will. That's how winning is done, indeed. It's a lesson not just of survival but of thriving, of taking the hits and still moving forward because life is a bout that goes beyond the final bell.

My fever raged as a child, the scarlet invader coursing through me, threatening to quench the young fire of my existence. But there she was, the guardian at the gate, holding back the darkness with a cool cloth and the promise of Dr. Dean's visit. The gentle hum of the television played counterpoint to the ragged rhythm of my breathing, cartoons flickering across the screen in shades of gray while my world burned with feverish color.

"Dr. Dean will be here soon, Bobby," she reassured, her voice the anchor in my delirium. "Just hold on."

And hold on I did because that's what we Quayles do—we endure. We aren't strangers to the precipice of despair nor are we unfamiliar with the climb back from its depths. I think of the countless others out there, lying on couches of their own, fighting unseen battles, and I feel a kinship with them, a shared thread in the tapestry of human struggle.

That's the story I'm writing now—not just my own but a chorus of voices that sing a hymn of resilience. It's a tale spun from hope's golden thread, woven through the fabric of a past that could have smothered us but instead made us stronger. With each word I write, I am stitching together the fragments of memory, crafting a legacy that might someday warm another soul caught in the chill of hardship.

"Thank you," I whisper, the gratitude spilling out for my mother, for life's harsh lessons, and for the strength that carried us through. I look around, seeing not the shadows of evening but the glow of dawn. Our luck, it seems, isn't found—it's forged in the fires of our will and the steel of our hearts. And so I write on, hopeful.

The beads of sweat on my forehead felt like a cascade, each drop a reminder of the fever's fierce grip. My mother's voice was a distant hum in the background, muffled by the heat enveloping me as I lay on that old, worn couch. The black-and-white cartoons flickered silently on the TV screen, their laughter and antics lost to my weary mind. With each labored breath, I felt myself slipping further from the living room from the sound of my mother's concerned phone call, from consciousness itself.

Then it happened—an ethereal drift into the unknown. It was a luminous tunnel, stretching out with an end that promised something beyond the pain and the delirium. A light so bright, so enveloping it was as if it reached inside me, tugging gently at the very essence of who I was. And there, within that embrace of pure white, a forest emerged around me, serene, and untouched.

A man appeared before me, his presence calming and familiar in a way that words could never capture. He knelt, locking eyes with me, and in those eyes, I found an ocean of understanding. "It's too soon, Bobby," he imparted with a voice that echoed through the trees, "you have a lot of work to do. Your father is with you. It's time to return." My eyelids fluttered open, the dream—or vision—receding like the tide, leaving only the echo of its message. And there he was, my father, standing over me with an expression I couldn't quite read. His visits were as scarce as rain in a drought, each one a moment etched in memory for its rarity rather than its warmth.

"How are you feeling?" he asked, his voice strangely gentle. I wanted to tell him about the tunnel, the light, the forest, but I knew our conversations were never meant for such depths. We shared a bloodline, yet the currents of our lives flowed in starkly different directions. As children, my sister and I had learned the harsh discipline of silence in the company of our godparents, where our father would take us. Those encounters were stiff, filled with unspoken questions and the weighty expectation of being seen and not heard. Even now, I wondered what my father thought as he watched me battle the fever, whether he saw beyond the illness to the son he barely knew.

Yet even in the shadow of his intermittent presence, I found a strange solace. Perhaps it was the nearness to something else, something profound that lingered just beyond my grasp in the wake of the feverish journey. There was an undeniable resilience within me, a hope that my father's unexpected visit signaled a turn in the tides of fortune.

Despite the arduous path life had laid before me, I understood that every trial, every tribulation, was but a steppingstone—a forging of character, a testament to the indomitable spirit inherited from my mother and, perhaps, even from the enigmatic figure of my father. And so I clung to the hope that sprouted from adversity. For if my mother's battles taught me anything, it was that even when life seems poised to break us, we can emerge stronger, fiercer, more alive. We may stumble and fall, but it is in the rising that we truly find ourselves.

"Better," I managed to whisper back to my father, offering him a faint smile. Better because I was still here, because I had returned from that brilliant light with a renewed sense of purpose. Better because, much like my mother, I was a fighter—a survivor destined to write my own story of triumph against all odds. In that moment, I didn't see the fading day or the encroaching night; I saw a canvas awaiting the colors of my will, my heart, and the unwavering belief that no matter how dire the circumstances, hope always finds a way to shine through.

The sun filtered through the canopy of leaves, casting a dappled dance of light and shadow on the forest floor. I could hear the laughter and banter of my friends as we navigated the edge of the ravine, our youthful energy undeterred by the sheer drop that loomed beside us. The Metroparks were our playground, a verdant escape from the concrete confines of our apartment complex, and on this day, we had discovered something new—a swing.

Not just any swing but a behemoth anchored to a sturdy oak, its long rope and wooden seat promising an unmatched thrill. With the boundless courage that only a twelve-year-old can muster, I stepped forward, my heart pounding in my chest as I reached for the rough texture of the rope. My fingers wrapped around it, feeling the fibers that held both promise and peril.

The oak seemed to beckon us, its ancient limbs outstretched like the arms of a wise elder daring us to test our mettle. The rope swing dangled there, an artifact from countless seasons past, its wood worn smooth by the hands of brave souls before us. We huddled at the edge of the ravine, the drop yawning below us, and gazed at that simple contraption as if it were a portal to another realm. Should we? Shouldn't we?

"Man, that looks old," one friend muttered, his voice tinged with the kind of trepidation I'd read about but never truly felt. I nodded, more out of social courtesy than agreement. Fear was a foreign language to me; I understood the concept, but it never quite translated in my heart. As a boy, this absence of fear often tipped the scales toward recklessness, sending me headlong into scrapes and bruises. But as I navigated the rocky terrain of life, that same void became a reservoir of courage, allowing me to leap where others might have balked.

"Let's just check it out," I suggested, approaching the tree with a feigned casualness, masking the adrenaline already beginning to course through my veins. We circled the swing warily, reaching out to touch the rope, testing its strength with tentative tugs. It was frayed, the strands of hemp unraveling slightly under our fingers, whispering secrets of countless storms weathered, of relentless cycles of freeze and thaw. Yet despite its battered appearance, it held firm beneath our experimental pulls.

"Looks fine to me," I said, a half-truth borne of desire rather than conviction. I hesitated for a moment, peering over the edge. The stream below was a silver ribbon threading through the rocks and earth, easily over a hundred feet down. The breath of the forest seemed to pause, waiting for my decision. In the stillness, I found clarity. This, right here, was a challenge. It was a test not just of courage but of trust—the kind that had been worn thin by broken promises and unspoken fears.

"Go for it, Bobby!" one of my friends called out, his voice a catalyst to action. With a deep breath that tasted like freedom, I pulled back on the swing, letting momentum gather before releasing myself into the air. Time slowed as I arced out over the ravine, the ground falling away, leaving me suspended between earth and sky. There was a split second at the apex where the world hushed, where I was nothing but a heartbeat and a breath, staring down the jaws of the ravine.

It was in that heartbeat that I felt alive—truly, vividly alive. Not just because of the adrenaline that surged through my veins but because I was making a choice. Despite everything, despite the bruises on my soul and the shadows of my past, I was choosing to soar. Gravity reclaimed me, pulling me back toward the safety of solid ground, and as my feet touched down, a laugh escaped my lips, pure and unburdened. It was the sound of resilience, of a spirit that refused to be caged by circumstance. As I handed off the swing to the next eager soul, my gaze lifted to the sky above, to the endless blue that whispered of possibilities and futures yet written.

"Did you see that?" I asked nobody in particular, the words spilling forth like a prayer of gratitude. In those moments, high above the rushing stream and jagged boulders, I glimpsed the shape of my life to come. It would be a tapestry of trials and triumphs, woven with the threads of hope my mother instilled in me. And as I stood there among friends, with the echo of the swing's flight still ringing in my ears, I knew that whatever lay ahead, I would face it head-on. Because if there's one thing I've learned from the towering oak and its daring swing, it's that taking a leap might just give you wings. And sometimes it's the very act of jumping that teaches you how to fly.

One by one, with hearts hammering against rib cages, we took turns on the swing. Each launch into the void brought screams that mingled with exhilaration and pure, unadulterated joy—a symphony of the living. The world blurred into streaks of green and brown as we arced out over the abyss, the rush of wind snatching away our breath, the very essence of being alive magnified in those fleeting seconds of flight. Back and forth, we flew, the ravine beneath us a gaping maw that could swallow us whole, yet somehow rendered impotent by our airborne defiance. I watched my friends, their faces alight with the kind of primal happiness that only comes from dancing with danger, and I couldn't help but feel a kinship with the generations who had swung here before us.

For what is existence if not a series of swings over the great ravines of life? We hang suspended between birth and death, joy and sorrow, soaring on the highs and recoiling from the lows. And here, on this swing, I was learning the art of balance—how to embrace the peaks without fearing the inevitable descent.

"All right, your turn again, Bobby!" they called, snapping me back from my reverie. As I grasped the rope, feeling the rough fibers bite into my palms, I knew that no matter how much time erodes the threads of our lives, we're all just seeking that moment of pure abandon—that second when we're neither rising nor falling but simply existing in the brilliant now.

"Here goes nothing," I murmured, stepping off the edge once more, ready to ride the pendulum of fate wherever it might swing. My hands clutched the rope with purpose, and I pushed off from the solid earth, propelling myself into that liberating arc over the deep ravine. Each pass toward the sky felt like an affirmation of the human spirit, a silent declaration that we are more than our fears, more than the fragile bodies that carry us.

"Go, Bobby! Farther!" my friends cheered, their voices a catalyst to my already daring nature. The sun was a spotlight on this stage of youthful bravado, and I was eager for my grand finale. With a force born of adrenaline and sheer will, I gave myself an extra shove, aiming to carve a wider swath across the open air to reach a little closer to the impossible. The world stopped, frozen in a moment of anticipation as I soared to the highest point of my jump. Then, with a deafening crack like thunder, the rope snapped. Then I was falling, falling, falling, my body hurtling toward the earth at a terrifying speed, my friends' screams and gasps drowned out by the rush of wind and my own pounding heart. But strangely, fear was absent, replaced by an eerie calmness that settled over me like a shroud.

Just before impact, everything shifted as if time slowed down. The ground rushing toward me seemed to blur and distort, and then…nothing. Instead of hitting solid rock or earth, I landed in a cradle of soft soil and gravel, my legs submerged in the cool water of the shallow stream. For a moment, all was still as I struggled to catch my breath against the weight of dirt pressing down on me.

"Are you okay?" my friends' panicked voices finally reached me through the haze. I was more than okay. Not a single scratch or bruise marked my skin, no blood to stain the crystal-clear water. In that moment, I felt invincible, untouchable. As if this was just another example of the universe conspiring to prove my mother right—that I was her lucky Mr. Magoo who always managed to escape unscathed.

With a wave to reassure my friends, I pulled myself out of the stream and began climbing back up to where we started. It wasn't until we were all safe and sound on top of the ravine that it hit me— this near-death experience could have ended very differently. And yet here we were, alive and laughing hysterically.

"Did you guys see that? I'm fine!" My voice trembled with awe and disbelief as we shared in the miracle of survival. And somewhere in the back of my mind, a voice whispered, "Not yet, Bobby," a reminder that my time had not yet come. But for now, I stood tall and proud, grateful for the second chance and the power to rise above fear and stand on my own two feet.

"Unbelievable," they muttered, shaking their heads as if trying to realign reality with the spectacle they'd just witnessed. In that moment, drenched and disheveled by the stream, I felt it—the indestructible thread of hope woven through the tapestry of my life. I couldn't know then how this resilience would shape my future, but I sensed its significance, a precursor to the many battles I would face and overcome.

"Let's head back," I suggested, my voice steady, my steps sure. "We've got more adventures ahead." And with that, we turned our backs on the broken swing on the ravine that had tried but failed to claim me, walking toward tomorrow, toward the rest of our lives.

"How is that even possible that he wasn't hurt?" they asked each other as they walked home.

*****

The wind whipped past my face as I pedaled furiously, the roof's edge approaching with the inevitability of time itself. My heart hammered in my chest; each beat a drumroll to the impending leap. I was fourteen and invincible, or so I thought. The bike's wheels left the shingles behind with a clatter, and for a brief, weightless moment, I flew. Then gravity reasserted itself, and I thudded into the grass below, the breath whooshing from my lungs. I lay there, staring at the sky, grinning like a lunatic. I'd done it—rode my bike off the roof on nothing but a dare.

"Mr. Magoo strikes again!" I muttered to myself, recalling my mother's nickname for me. I stood up, gazing at the mangled bike next to me, evidence of my daring stunt. My friends were in awe, unable to believe that I had actually pulled it off.

That wasn't the only high-stakes game I played with fate. Behind our house stood a 150-foot-tall electrical tower, its lattice structure a siren call to my sense of adventure. Up I would climb, hand over hand, the metal cold and unyielding against my palms, higher and higher until the world below became a patchwork quilt of mundane concerns. At the top, the air vibrated with the hum of power coursing through the lines, a sound you could feel in your bones. I'd lean out, just far enough to feel the electric thrum tickle my fingertips and carve "B.Q." into the steel.

"Your mom wants you to get down!" the neighborhood kids would yell up to me.

I'd glance down, their figures small and distorted by the distance, and respond in the universal language of rebellious youth—a defiant arc of urine and an upraised middle finger. They'd scatter, squealing, as I laughed and yelled, "Watch out for yellow rain!" King of my concrete jungle.

But perhaps the most thrilling of my youthful escapades involved the freight trains that rumbled by our neighborhood. I'd wait for the slow chug of the wheels, then run alongside before hoisting myself up with a grunt. Once aboard, I'd sit back and enjoy the ride, the landscape sliding by in a blur of greens and browns. It was a shortcut to my girlfriend's house, a way to show up with a story, a badge of my courage—or so I liked to think.

"Wow, Bobby, you're crazy!" she'd exclaim, her eyes wide with a mix of admiration and concern.

"Yeah, well, that's me," I'd say, puffing up a bit with pride.

Then came the day when the train didn't just lumber—it lurched, picking up speed with an urgency I hadn't anticipated. My heart skipped. This wasn't the leisurely pace that I was used to; this was something else entirely. The bridge loomed ahead, a long stretch of nothing but air and water beneath. I had to make a choice and fast.

"Stay calm," I whispered to myself, steadying my breathing. I crouched, ready to roll if I needed to disembark in a hurry, every muscle tensed for action.

"Control," I reminded myself. "You've got this."

The train roared onward and I with it, into the unknown. But I was no stranger to fear, to danger, to the unexpected twists life throws your way. With every challenge, I found another piece of myself—a stubborn hope, a resilience as tough as the steel I once scaled.

Let's see where this goes, I mused, a faint smile touching my lips, even as the adrenaline surged within me. The bridge was approaching, but so was my future—unwritten, uncertain, but entirely mine to shape.

The train was a metal beast, unrelenting in its newfound speed, its wheels thundering against the tracks with a ferocity that sent shivers down my spine. The bridge ended, and the landscape opened up before me, revealing an ominous body of water that promised a temporary escape. Frantic thoughts rattled my brain as the pond neared, my heart pounding in rhythm with the clattering cars.

"Jump," I urged myself, the word more a lifeline than a command. And so I did. My body arced through the air, arms flailing for balance I couldn't find, gravity pulling me down to an abrupt, squelching halt. It wasn't water that enveloped me but a greasy black muck—a stinking, viscous pit that clung to me like a second skin.

Coughing, retching, I stumbled onto the gravel road, each step heavy with the weight of the fetid sludge. The walk home was torturous, the odor a constant companion that forced bile into my throat every few paces.

Those solitary moments, trudging along with the stench of failure clinging to me, could have been the end of another chapter marked by recklessness. But they weren't.

My mother, a woman who'd seen her fair share of hardship, had always sought better for us. She moved us away from the city's chaos to the quiet of the suburbs, not realizing the silence would be my undoing. In the city, the advanced classes had kept my mind engaged, racing to keep up with the barrage of information. In the suburbs, however, I found myself adrift in a sea of ennui, the curriculum too slow to contain my restless thoughts.

Then tragedy struck just a street over, tearing through our quiet neighborhood like a tornado. It struck close to home, in the form of a deranged criminal who had been silently observing our daily routines. Each morning, we gathered at the bus stop, smoking and chatting before school. Steve, my friend from down the block, would join us after walking along the railroad tracks behind his house to meet our other friend, Mike, at his house before continuing to the bus stop. But on this fateful day, they never appeared.

As I walked past Mike's house toward the bus stop, I heard gunshots echoing from behind me but brushed it off as hunters in the nearby woods. Then, as I continued walking to the bus stop, emergency vehicles with flashing lights and blaring sirens sped past me, stopping in front of Mike's house. Confused and curious, I continued on my way until I realized what had happened.

The deranged boyfriend of Mike's older sister had arrived in a murderous rage that morning. He held Steve and Mike at gunpoint, demanding entry into the house before ultimately ordering them to leave or face death. In an act of desperation, they ran to Steve's house to call for help while I unknowingly walked by in the front.

But by then, it was too late. The murderer had taken out his twisted anger on Mike's entire family—first killing his parents as they lay in bed and then taking his sister's life before finally ending his own. A senseless tragedy had occurred right under our noses.

In the aftermath of shock and sorrow, a dangerous thrill-seeking part of me began to stir, desperate for anything to break the monotony. Yet amid all the chaos, a small spark of ambition remained within me—refusing to be snuffed out by tragedy.

"Think, Bobby, there's got to be more to life than this," I'd tell myself.

And there was. This realization became my salvation. At sixteen, two years ahead of schedule, with the school's reluctant blessing, I cast off the chains of traditional education to explore the vast unknown that lay beyond the classroom walls.

Reflecting on these turns of fate, I understand now that resilience isn't just about getting back up; it's about seeking new paths when the old ones lead you astray. It's about hope, the kind that lights a fire in your belly and propels you forward, even when you're covered in muck and life reeks of rotten eggs.

As I walked, the sun dipped lower, painting the sky in shades of amber and gold. A gentle breeze whispered promises through the trees, and I listened, knowing that despite the setbacks, despite the filth, I was moving toward something greater. Because sometimes, you have to fall into the muck to find your way out of the darkness and into the light.

CHAPTER 4

A New Future Awaits

The last echoes of "Pomp and Circumstance" still played in the corners of my mind as I cast a line into the calm waters of the river that wound through the Metroparks. The ripples from the bait's entry whispered to me of freedom, a soft promise that life was now mine to steer. With school behind me, every day unfolded like an unwritten page, crisp and beckoning under summer's gaze.

I sat there on the banks, often alone, feeling the world stretch out before me, vast and uncharted. My friends, bound by routines of work and classes, followed timeworn paths while I lingered under the sun, pondering the roads less traveled. In those solitary hours, punctuated only by the distant rumble of trains jostling over bridges, I found comfort in reflection. The very bridges that trembled with the weight of passing trains were once under my feet, a blur of motion as I rode atop them, hurtling toward destinations unknown.

Luck had always been a peculiar companion of mine, showing up in moments when hope seemed thin. We weren't well-off, my family and I, so luxuries like concert tickets to see rock legends—Billy Joel topping the list of favorites—were beyond our means. But necessity is the mother of invention, and I became a maestro at the art of winning radio contests. The push-button phone was my instrument, my fingers nimble dancers across its numbered stage. The anticipation built as the DJ's voice crackled through the speaker, ready to announce the magic number. A deep breath, then a flurry of movement, digits pressing down in rapid succession.

"Congratulations! You're caller number nine!" the voice would say, elation flooding through the line. It became a ritual, a game of timing and precision that brought music to my ears—quite literally. A thrill surged each time I claimed victory, snagging those coveted tickets against all odds.

But as it goes with games of chance, rules change to even the playing field. The radio stations caught on to my streak and introduced limitations—a winner only once per month per household. Yet where some saw a roadblock, I saw a detour. I enlisted friends' names and addresses, a workaround that kept the concerts within reach. It was a testament to my resourcefulness, a knack for navigating around life's little hurdles.

On a sunny day in early spring, my sister, Deborah or Deb as I call her, emerged from her bedroom with a determined look on her face. At fourteen years old, she was in the throes of a teenage obsession with Rick Springfield, much like every other girl her age. Her birthday was just around the corner, at the end of March, and it just so happened that Rick Springfield would be performing in our area around the same time. The local radio stations were buzzing with excitement, giving away tickets to lucky callers.

As she walked past me with a disdainful sneer, typical of teenage siblings, the DJ's voice boomed through the speakers: "Be caller number 12 and win front row seats to see Rick Springfield!"

Without hesitation, I sauntered over to the phone, picked it up at precisely the right moment, dialed the number, and heard it ring on the other end. With a sly grin, I handed the phone over to my skeptical sister.

"Who is this?" she asked suspiciously.

I replied nonchalantly, "It's WMMS, and you just won tickets to see Rick Springfield. Happy birthday!"

In disbelief, she answered the phone and gave me a knowing look that said she wasn't falling for my trick. But then we heard the DJ's booming voice exclaiming, "Congratulations! You're going to see Rick Springfield!"

My sister's expression changed to one of shock and joy as she exclaimed, "Oh my gosh! WMMS! Thank you so much!"

As I sat by the river, these memories mingled with the hum of nature, a symphony of past and present. The solitude fed my introspection, fueling dreams not yet dreamt. Each cast line was a question sent forth into the universe, each tug at the rod an answer pending. Life was a canvas, and I held the brush, ready to paint my destiny with broad strokes of resilience and hope.

And so amid the dance of dragonflies and the rustle of leaves, I found strength in the waiting, in the patience required to reel in whatever fortunes lay beneath the surface. There was a sense of knowing, a certainty that luck was my ally, and that the next big catch, the next serendipitous pull, was just beyond the horizon.

I was lucky to have a group of friends who were always up for adventure, even if it often got us in trouble. Greg, Kevin, and Steve were my partners in crime, and we spent countless hours roaming the neighborhood looking for mischief to get into.

At the time, I considered Greg to be my closest friend. But as I reflect on our relationship, I realize that he wasn't the most reliable or genuine companion. Despite his small stature and lean frame, there was a mischievous spark in his eyes that always kept me on edge. Our bond formed over late nights spent playing video games and mutual disdain for school. It didn't hurt that our parents were also close friends, making it seem like our friendship was predestined. However, I must admit one of the main reasons I enjoyed hanging out with him was his younger sister, with whom I would sneak off to make out during our sleepovers.

Kevin was the sidekick of our group. He was short for a boy at the time, with long hair that always seemed to be in his face. He wasn't as daring as Greg or me, but he always had our backs and was up for anything.

Steve lived just down the street from me and became part of our group when we were around thirteen years old. He was taller than all of us and had a laid-back personality that balanced out our rowdiness perfectly. We often hung out at his house, playing video games or watching movies.

Together, we were known as the troublemakers of the neighborhood. We would often terrorize the streets by toilet-papering yards, egging houses, and playing pranks on unsuspecting neighbors. It wasn't uncommon for us to stay out late into the night, causing mayhem.

On a warm summer day, we set out to build a fort in the lush forest behind our suburban development. The sun shone high in the sky as we carefully stacked wooden pallets and scraps of wood to create our hideaway. Everything went smoothly until the sun began its descent, casting a chilly breeze through the trees.

Realizing that the temperature was dropping rapidly, we decided to start a campfire to keep warm. But as soon as we lit the fire, the dry leaves and grass surrounding our fort ignited as well, flames erupted with startling speed, despite our efforts to contain it with stones.

To make matters worse, we had built our fire at the base of a tree that served as one wall of our fort. The flames quickly climbed up its trunk, engulfing our creation and threatening to spread further into the forest.

Panicked and terrified, we ran toward the nearest house, pounding on the door with urgency. An older man, probably in his sixties or seventies, appeared, and we pleaded for him to call 911 as we pointed frantically at the forest across the street from his home.

As he dialed for help, the man must have realized that it was us who had started the fire—our clothes were smudged with ash and we smelled strongly of smoke. "Stay right there," he commanded before disappearing back into his home.

But by the time he returned, we were already sprinting down the road toward safety, nearly a quarter mile away. With bated breath, we watched as the fire department arrived just in time to extinguish the flames before they could do any major damage.

Once the danger had passed and our hearts had stopped racing, we were relieved that no one was hurt and there was minimal harm done. It was a lesson learned—never underestimate the power of nature and always be cautious when playing with fire.

The summer sun beat down on us with a ferocity that could fry an egg on the sidewalk, but we had found our sanctuary beneath the railroad bridges of my hometown, Berea. The trestles, as we called them, were like the ribs of some giant concrete beast, offering shade and secrecy from the world above. In that hidden realm, we carved out a place for ourselves, a no-man's-land where the rules of suburbia didn't apply.

I can still taste the bitter tang of cigarette smoke mingling with the sweet burn of cheap whiskey stolen from liquor cabinets. We would pass a joint around, its ember glowing against the dim backdrop of our cave-like hideout. Sometimes, in the audacity of youth, we'd hurl snowballs at passing cars below, our laughter echoing off the walls as drivers cursed into the void, unaware of the band of misfits perched above.

There was an undeniable thrill in those moments of rebellion, a sense of invincibility that only the ignorance of adolescence can provide. It was foolishness, yes, but it was also freedom—the kind that makes you believe you're the master of your own destiny, even when you're just a kid throwing water balloons and snowballs at the world.

Away from my comrades-in-mischief, solitude became my companion. My hands, ever restless, sought new projects. One sweltering afternoon, I decided the backyard needed a pond. With nothing but a shovel and youthful determination, I set to work. The earth gave way beneath my efforts, each shovelful a small victory. The finished result was less a pond and more a testament to boredom—a muddy pit that earned me nothing but a scolding for ruining the lawn. But oh how my imagination had reveled in the doing!

Winter brought its own brand of restlessness. Surveying the snow-blanketed landscape, inspiration struck like lightning. From the top of the garage, I envisioned a sled run grander than any other. I piled snow high, sculpting curves and banking turns, a white-knuckle track that would make any amusement park proud. The fence of our unsuspecting neighbor formed a perfect boundary, unwittingly contributing to my makeshift luge with its starting point at the peak of the garage.

"Mom, you've got to try this," I urged, my breath visible in the frosty air as I pointed at the stairs of ice leading to the top of the garage. I had put a layer of gravel on each step for traction.

Elaine, my mother, a woman whose life had been tougher than most, eyed the construction with apprehension. Yet there was a flicker of something wild in her gaze—a spark reignited from days long past. With courage I hadn't known she possessed, she climbed to the summit of my creation. The sled, a flimsy plastic disk, awaited her command.

"Are you sure about this?" she asked, the doubt evident in her voice.

"Absolutely," I assured her, masking my own uncertainty with bravado.

With a push, she descended, picking up speed, a streak of color against the white canvas. The sled careened, hugged the turn, and shot out into the open expanse of the yard. Her laughter rang clear and pure, a sound that stitched itself into the fabric of my memory. She emerged from the ride, wide-eyed and breathless, exhilarated by the unexpected adventure.

"Again!" she exclaimed, her spirit alight with a joy I hadn't seen in years. My younger sister, Deb, joined in the delight, and together they hurtled down the makeshift luge. The wind whipped through their hair, and their laughter echoed through the air as they picked up speed. The icy snow sprayed up around them, soaking their clothes and leaving them chilled to the bone. But they couldn't stop, not until they reached the bottom and collapsed onto the snow, panting and exhilarated from their wild ride.

In those moments, both brazen and quiet, I learned the essence of what it means to truly live. It wasn't about the mischief or the escapades; it was the unbridled joy of creating, of experiencing, of daring to make something out of nothing. My path was not yet clear, but I was learning to embrace the journey, to trust in the luck that seemed to follow me, and to seize every opportunity to fill my days with stories worth telling.

And as I reflect now, with the wisdom of years gently settling upon my shoulders, I see how each act of defiance, each project embarked upon, was a step toward understanding myself. Those days of freedom and independence, they were the building blocks of the man I am today. They taught me resilience, ignited hope, and fanned the flames of luck that have burned steadily through the trials of life.

I sat cross-legged and contemplative under the gnarled apple trees that had been silent witnesses to much of my youth. The grass beneath us was a wild sea of green, crested with dandelions gone to seed, whispering against the fabric of our jeans as if urging us to take notice of the passing time.

There, in the dappled shade, with the sun playing hide and seek through the leaves, I felt a strange serenity wash over me—a pause in the relentless march of life. Bonnie, my loyal pet rabbit, hopped contentedly within her makeshift enclosure at the tree's base. She nibbled on the tender grass, every now and then lifting her head to sniff at the fallen fruit, embodying a simple pleasure that seemed so elusive to us at that moment.

The smell of summer was in the air, a mix of overripe apples and fresh-cut grass—a scent that always seemed to stir up the entrepreneur within me. My friends and I were lounging in the backyard, our conversation lazily circling around one topic: money. We needed it for the essentials of teenage life—beers, dates, and enough green to keep the good times rolling.

I stretched out my legs, brushing the grass clippings off my jeans, eyes scanning the horizon for inspiration. It wasn't as if I hadn't been down this road before. That summer had seen me knee-deep in fields, hands cautiously guiding wild snakes into sacks. The hiss and slither of scales had become oddly comforting sounds as I traded them in at the local pet store. On quieter days, the soft scratching of mice and hamsters I bred filled the silence of my room, each tiny creature a coin in my makeshift piggy bank.

"Guys, there's always something," I mused aloud, my mind sifting through possibilities like panning for gold. "You just gotta know where to look."

And look I did. Back when winter's chill still bit at our heels, old Mr. Jenkins, the farmer with land adjoining ours, had made me an interesting offer. His voice, rough from years of shouting over tractor engines, still echoed in my memory, "Bobby, you get me those praying mantis eggs, and I'll give you fifty dollars a bucket."

He had taken the time to show me how to spot the frothy masses clinging to tree branches, tiny fortresses of life waiting to erupt. Each one was a potential gold mine. "Cheapest insecticide nature ever cooked up," he'd said, his wrinkled face breaking into a grin. "Better than any chemical those big companies will sell ya."

Luck, it seemed, didn't just find me. I had a knack for seeking it out, for coaxing it from the underbrush or the branches of trees. I remember thinking how odd it was, the notion of farming insects, but then again, that's what life often boils down to—finding value in the unexpected.

I cradled the two heavy buckets, their contents a fortune in tiny, spherical capsules of life. The farmer's eyes had twinkled with a kind of rural wisdom as he spoke of the praying mantises, nature's little soldiers against pests. Fifty dollars a bucket was a small price for him but a windfall for me. I was set to trek across the fields to his farmstead when Mom called out, reminding me of our weekend plans. My heart sank a notch; the eggs couldn't be left unattended.

"Hide 'em somewhere safe," she suggested, busy packing for our trip. So into my closet went the precious cargo, shrouded in darkness and secrecy, safe from thieving hands. I never considered the warmth of an indoor summer would act as an incubator.

We returned on Sunday to a spectacle that would have enthralled any entomologist. A biblical exodus of praying mantises had emerged, turning my room into a writhing nursery. They clung to my posters, my bedspread, even dangled from the ceiling light like odd tinsel. It was awe-inspiring and horrifying in equal measure. With the vacuum hose in hand, I became an unwilling Pied Piper, ushering thousands of tiny lives back into the wild. To this day, our house is known for its ever-vigilant insect guardians patrolling the garden boundaries, descendants of my unintended hatchery.

"Hey, Bobby, you daydreaming on us again?" one of my friends called out, snapping me back to the present.

"Just thinking about last winter," I replied, gaze drifting to the apple tree limbs above, laden with the promise of fruit—and perhaps other profitable harvests. "Remember those mantis eggs?"

Laughter bubbled up from our circle, a shared memory of my bedroom turned accidental insect nursery. But there was admiration there, too, in their teasing. They knew that when it came to making a dollar, I could pull opportunity out of thin air—or thick foliage, as it were.

"Always hustling," another chimed in with a chuckle, shaking his head.

That's just it, though. Life's a hustle—a series of problems to be solved, opportunities to be grabbed. And I realized, sitting there, surrounded by my friends and the dappled shade of the apple trees, that every quirky moneymaking scheme was more than just quick cash. It was the groundwork for the resilience that would define my life.

"Come on, let's keep brainstorming," I urged, feeling the spark of hope that always flared when a plan began to take shape. It was the same hope that guided my steps, that whispered of better things to come if only I had the courage to reach out and seize them.

"Man, we need cash," muttered one of my friends, breaking the silence that had settled over us. We were a small band of dreamers and schemers, bound by our shared restlessness and the unspoken understanding that life was calling us to something more—something beyond the haze of our aimless summers.

We each took turns drawing from the joint that was making its ritualistic round, its embers glowing brighter with each inhale. As the smoke curled upward, joining the fragmented light above, ideas began to spark within the fertile ground of my mind.

"Maybe we could do odd jobs around the neighborhood," someone suggested halfheartedly, but it held no allure. No, the ambition burning within me sought a grander stage than manicured lawns and whitewashed fences.

"Or sell stuff at the flea market," another added, but the thought fizzled out as quickly as it came, lost in the collective exhale of disinterest.

I felt the weight of Bonnie's tranquil gaze upon me, her innocent eyes a stark contrast to the whirlwind of thoughts storming through my head. The problem wasn't just about getting money—it was about finding a way to live vibrantly, to seize the days ahead with both hands and mold them into something memorable.

"There has to be something more we can do," I mused aloud, watching the smoke curl upward, dissipating into nothing—much like our half-baked schemes for quick cash. Flashes of lawn mowers and fast-food uniforms flickered through my thoughts, but they were mere shadows of an idea not yet fully formed.

Then it struck, a spark in the dusk of indecision. "The county fair!" I exclaimed, sitting bolt upright, the joint momentarily forgotten between my fingers. It was more than an event; it was an opportunity, a cavalcade of chances bustling into town. "I bet we could snag some jobs there."

The suggestion was met with a spark of enthusiasm, the first real flicker of excitement since we'd settled under the apple trees' watchful canopy. It was a plan with legs, with movement; it promised adventure.

"Let's check it out," I declared, feeling the pull of destiny—or perhaps just the thrill of the unknown.

As we rose from our circle, leaving behind the indentations of our presence in the long grass, I glanced back at Bonnie. She was still munching away, blissfully unaware of the cogs turning in our human minds. Yet in her simplicity, she was a reminder of life's constant motion—the ebb and flow that brings change, growth, and sometimes the answer to an unasked question.

In many ways, that summer distilled who I was—a young man not afraid to get his hands dirty, to walk the less trodden path if it meant finding success in its hidden corners. It was the beginning of something greater, the first threads of a larger story being woven, one that spoke of determination, innovation, and the kind of luck that comes to those willing to look for it.

"Whatever we decide," I said, standing up and stretching, "we're going to make it work. We always do." With a smile, I looked down at Bonnie, still content in her pen, and thought how life, much like my rabbit, sometimes required a gentle hand and the patience to wait for the right moment to hop toward your next adventure.

The fair—it was a place of magic and noise, of color and light, where fortunes could turn on the toss of a ring or the roll of a ball. It was where hope was packaged in bright balloons and the promise of adventure beckoned from every stall. My friends, though skeptical, saw the eagerness in my eyes and knew better than to doubt the gut instincts that so often led us down paths less traveled.

"Let's check it out," I said, the words laced with the potential of what could be. Handing off the smoldering joint to a friend, I stood up, feeling the familiar surge of determination. This was it, another chapter waiting to be written, another anecdote for the book of my life that would one day tell a tale of perseverance and the sweet serendipity that followed those who dared to chase it.

That summer of '82 marked the beginning of a series of events that would shape the course of my life. Each decision, each chance taken, was a thread woven into the tapestry of my story—a narrative etched with resilience, hope, and a stroke of luck that always seemed to find me when I needed it most.

As I reflect on those days, with their brash decisions and bold dreams, I can't help but smile at the journey. It taught me that sometimes, you have to create your own tide, ride it out, and trust that wherever it takes you, it's exactly where you're meant to be.

The morning sun had barely begun to gild the tips of the tents when we arrived at the fairgrounds, a place transformed almost overnight from an empty field to a burgeoning hive of activity. We walked through the gates with purpose, our sneakers crunching on the gravel like a promise underfoot. Each step was a march toward independence, a chance to put some honest sweat into the world and reap the rewards.

"Let's split up," I suggested to my friends, "cover more ground that way." With nods of agreement, we dispersed amid the clamor of metal clanging and the smell of sawdust and fried food beginning to mingle in the air.

I found myself drawn to where the bumper cars were being assembled, a metallic skeleton yearning for life. A man with a handlebar mustache, sleeves rolled high over his tanned forearms, beckoned me over. "Need a hand?" I called out, not waiting for an invitation. He sized me up, nodded, and put me to work. The task was simple yet gratifying—fitting pieces together, wrenching bolts tight, becoming part of something larger than myself.

Ten hours passed like a dream of labor and camaraderie. My muscles ached, but it was the sweet pain of accomplishment. When the man handed each of us two crisp twenty-dollar bills, it felt like holding a treasure trove. That money wasn't just currency; it was freedom, possibilities, a summer stretching out before us ripe with potential.

"Life is good," I murmured, pocketing the bills, the weight of them a comforting assurance against the fabric.

The next day dawned with the same sense of possibility. We returned to the fairgrounds eager for more work, our pockets noticeably heavier from the previous day's efforts. The fair was taking shape now, vibrant and chaotic, as workers scurried about like a colony of bees, each knowing their role in this dance of creation.

"*Hey, you lookin' fer work, boooy?!*" The voice cut through the din, a rasp seasoned with years of shouting to be heard over carnival music. I turned to see a carny motioning toward me, his grin wide and gap-toothed.

"Sure am," I replied, stepping closer. There was something about his demeanor, missing teeth and all, that seemed to embody the spirit of the fair itself—a little rough around the edges but full of life and stories.

"Good," he said, nodding in approval. "Got plenty to do 'round here."

As I followed him to my next task, I felt the stirrings of pride within me. It wasn't just about making money anymore, though that was certainly a driving force. It was about proving to myself that I could carve out a niche in this world, that I could stand on my own two feet and face whatever challenges came my way. With every booth erected, every nail hammered, I was building more than just the fair—I was constructing the foundation of my future.

And somewhere, in the back of my mind, a hopeful thought took root: maybe luck was something you made for yourself, with your own hands, in places just like this.

The sun had already climbed high by the time I settled into my new role at the fair. The carny, a wizened old man with more stories etched in his wrinkles than years I had been alive, was my mentor for the day. He gestured toward the game booth, its vibrant colors clashing joyously against the blue sky.

"All right, boy," he said, scratching his stubbled chin. "You see this here game? Gonna teach you the ropes—literally."

I nodded, eager to learn another way to pad my pockets. Money was freedom, and I was chasing it with the fervor of a man on fire. The carny demonstrated the technique required to stand a glass bottle upright using a pole with a plastic ring tied to the end of a rope. It looked simple enough when he did it, but my first few attempts were clumsy, the bottle tipping defiantly each time.

"Easy does it," he coached, a patient twinkle in his eye. "It's all in the wrist and a gentle touch."

Three days came and went, filled with practice and persistence. My hands learned the weight of the pole, the tension in the rope, and the balance point of the bottles. I became familiar with the feel of waxed wood beneath my fingers and the satisfying clink of success as the glass stood proud and tall.

"Making it look easy is what brings 'em in," the carny revealed, counting out a quarter for each dollar brought in as my share of the takings. "And, kid, you've got sales in your blood."

The fair became my kingdom and the game my throne. People crowded around, their eyes alight with challenge as I deftly maneuvered bottle after bottle. Their excitement turned to amazement, then determination as they handed over dollars to try their luck. And I, the orchestrator of their amusement, felt a rush every time the coins clicked against each other, adding up to my newfound wealth.

The sun was dipping low, throwing a kaleidoscope of oranges and purples across the fairground sky as I flicked my wrist with precision, standing another bottle upright. The crowd around my game booth murmured in appreciation—some with suspicion, others with the itch to try their luck. I had found my rhythm, a dance of showmanship that seemed to draw people in like moths to a flame.

"Hey there, cutie pie, would you like some information about the army?"

The voice cut through the hum of the midway, sharp and sweet. I glanced up, and for a moment, it felt like the world tilted on its axis.

Two incredibly beautiful girls stood before me, resplendent in crisp army uniforms, their smiles bright and inviting. They had an air of confidence and bodies that could easily command the attention of any young man, myself included.

"You two are in the army? Sign me up!" I blurted out before my brain could catch up with the audacity of my words. Their laughter was a melody that washed over me, filling me with a sense of possibility I hadn't known was missing.

But as they handed me the brochure, reality settled back in—a gentle reminder that I was here, at this fair, not as a soldier but as a purveyor of amusement, a master of this deceivingly simple game. My heart raced, though, not from the game or the hustle but from the sudden infusion of new dreams being whispered into my ear by fate herself.

With one last attempt at bravado, I asked for their numbers, fully expecting the polite rebuff that followed. Yet even in rejection, there was something affirming. It was a brush with life outside my own, a peek beyond the fence of my current existence.

In just five days, I'd amassed a small fortune—over $4,000 flowed through that booth, and a sweet $1,000 landed in my pocket. I couldn't believe it. I held the money, crisp and promising, feeling like Midas himself.

"Son," the carny implored, his voice husky with sincerity, "you're a natural. Ever think about hitting the road with us? I'll give you 35 cents on the dollar."

Temptation flickered, a siren's call to the unknown. But a glance at his weather-beaten face, and thoughts of my own kin waiting back home anchored me. I knew I wanted more than the transient life of a carny, no matter how sweet the offer.

"Thanks but no thanks," I replied firmly. "Got other plans brewing."

He nodded, understanding or perhaps disappointed—I couldn't tell. As I walked away from the fair that final night, pockets heavy and heart full, I didn't realize that fate had already laid her cards on the table. There, amid the laughter and the lights, a seed had been planted—one that would grow into a life I never imagined possible.

The resilience of those days, the unwavering hope in the face of uncertainty, and the self-made luck I carried with me—it was all part of a greater design. A design that, looking back now, was as clear as the bottles I stood up with such practiced ease.

That night, as I counted my earnings, the faces of those two girls lingered in my mind. They were sirens of a future unknown, messengers of opportunity. They weren't soldiers themselves, as I later discovered—just college girls playing a role. But they had unwittingly enlisted me into a broader spectrum of thought, opening doors in my mind that I hadn't realized were there to be opened.

As the day faded and the lights of the fair began to twinkle against the night, I felt a profound sense of gratitude—grateful for the game that showed me skill could be more than a trick of the hand, for the chance encounters that shaped my path, and for the ever-present undercurrent of luck that seemed to guide me when I needed it most.

The next day, the recruiter's knock on the door wasn't just a simple follow-up—it was the sound of destiny tapping at my doorstep. Each knock echoed with a sense of resilience and hope, reflecting on the journey that had brought me to this moment and the challenges I would face in the future. My unwavering belief in the serendipity of life in how unexpected turns can lead us to where we're meant to be once again proved true.

It had been about six months since I first met with the army recruiter. Those months seemed to fly by in a blur, filled with both excitement and anxiety for my new path serving my country. As I said goodbye to my friends during that time, our individual paths began to diverge as we approached adulthood. Greg, my closest friend, seemed especially upset about my departure. "You're abandoning me," he would say in frustration, his words causing a sharp pang in my heart. But deep down, I knew this was something I needed to do for myself and my future. Looking back now, I realize that he wasn't really a good friend after all—but that's a story best left untold.

And then, finally, the fateful day arrived—the relentless shrill of the alarm pierced through the predawn silence, jolting me awake from a restless sleep filled with dreams tinted with shades of olive drab and adventure. For a moment, I lay there in bed, heart pounding with adrenaline as reality slowly seeped in through the grogginess—that stubborn fog that clings onto you like a heavy weight. It was no ordinary day; it was March 17, 1983—St. Patrick's Day. But for me, it held no connotations of parades or revelry. Instead, it marked the day when my life would take an unexpected turn on an axis of profound change.

Swinging my legs off the bed, I felt the chill of the floorboards against my bare feet, a stark reminder that I was stepping into something much bigger than myself. I dressed silently amid the somber shadows, my movements deliberate, each second ticking by like a metronome set to the beat of my escalating pulse. My clothes felt foreign, as though I was trying on a character in a play—one I was about to live out for real.

Downstairs, the streets were already coming to life, the sounds of celebration a stark contrast to the solemnity of my mother's face as she watched me gulp down a hurried breakfast. Her reluctant consent still hung in the air, heavy and unspoken. I saw the worry etched in the lines of her brow, the raw fear that only a mother can feel as she watches her child march off to an uncertain destiny. Yet beneath it all was a glimmer of pride—a silent acknowledgment of the resilience I'd shown throughout my life.

"Take care of yourself," she murmured, the words caught somewhere between a whisper and a plea. I nodded, unable to trust my voice, and shouldered my bag. The weight of it seemed to anchor me, a physical manifestation of the gravity of my decision.

Stepping out into the brisk morning, I was greeted by the cacophony of St. Patrick's Day festivities. The streets were awash with green, throngs of merrymakers lost in the revelry of the holiday. Among them, I moved like a ghost, unnoticed, my own path taking me away from the conviviality and toward the bus terminal.

I arrived at the station to find it buzzing with activity, a hive of travelers each bound for different corners of the world. But there was only one destination on my ticket: Fort Jackson, South Carolina. Sitting on that cold metal bench, waiting for my bus to be called, I felt the tendrils of fear and excitement intertwine within me, a dance of contrasting emotions. I was leaving behind everything familiar, venturing into a future fraught with challenges and possibilities.

As the bus rolled into view, my heartbeat quickened. This was it—the threshold between what had been and what was yet to come. Climbing aboard, I found a window seat, pressing my forehead against the cool glass as we pulled away. The city receded into the distance, becoming nothing more than a patchwork of memories seen through the fading mist of the morning.

I thought of the fairgrounds, the sound of laughter, the thrill of the game, and those two girls in army uniforms who had knowingly nudged me onto this path. They were the catalysts, their brochures now a bridge to this very moment. And as the bus hummed along the highway, I allowed myself to imagine the person I might become—someone shaped by discipline, strengthened by trials, and perhaps, just maybe, someone who could make a difference.

The journey ahead was veiled in uncertainty, but my spirit was buoyant with hope. Life had a way of throwing curveballs, and I'd learned to swing, even when the pitch was unexpected. Maybe it was luck that had guided me here or maybe it was something else—something woven into the very fabric of who I was. But either way, I was ready to embrace whatever lay ahead because resilience isn't just about surviving; it's about thriving against the odds.

And so with the road stretching out before me like the first page of a new chapter, I leaned back in my seat, a smile tugging at the corner of my lips. I was terrified, yes, but thrilled at the prospect of becoming the architect of my own fate.

CHAPTER 5

A PROMISING CAREER

The first glimpse of Fort Jackson materialized like a mirage against the South Carolina heat, its storied grounds promising commencement, challenge, and change. We had arrived, the latest shipment of eager souls ready to be forged into something more than we were. The bus wheezed to a stop, exhaling us into the care of the military's embrace, and there they stood: the so-called "cattle cars" awaiting our boarding. These rugged, open-air transports bore no luxury, their benches hard and unforgiving, the metal skeleton vibrating with untold histories of transformation. I hoisted myself up, the weight of my duffel bag a sudden reminder of the gravity of this journey. As the cattle car lurched forward, I steadied myself, my hand gripping cold steel, feeling every jolt and bump along the unpaved paths that cut through dense forests like arteries of discipline. These vehicles weren't designed for comfort; they were vessels of utility, delivering us to the crucible where boys became soldiers.

Silence hung heavy among us trainees, but it was the hushed tones of the accompanying drill sergeants that carried an ominous weight. Their quiet was not born of peace but of the calm before a storm. In those days, "wall-to-wall counseling" wasn't just a phrase—it was a harsh reality for those who stepped out of line. The mere thought of being taken aside by these hardened mentors for a physical reckoning made my stomach churn. Yet somewhere within me, a spark of defiance kindled. If this was the rite of passage, then I would meet it head-on.

"Remember why you're here," I murmured to myself, a mantra against the brewing fear. My mind cast back to the family I had left behind—to my sister's unwavering gaze as she stood by my side, her belief in me a silent bastion against doubt; to my mother, Elaine, whose life of sacrifices and uncomplaining endurance had instilled in me a sense of purpose and grit. As the cattle car trundled on, I felt the eyes of Sergeant Martinez on us. She was tough, no question, but beneath that exterior lay a reservoir of empathy. Her brand of leadership was one that inspired rather than intimidated, even in silence. And then there was Greg, his humor a lifeline in dark times, reminding me that even in the midst of trial, there could be a glimmer of lightness.

"Combat doesn't care if you're comfortable," I reasoned, shifting to find a less punishing angle against the wooden bench. "And neither does life." It was a lesson I'd learned well before this moment and one I'd undoubtedly face again. But the anticipation of what lay ahead couldn't overshadow the deep-seated resilience that I, like so many before me, carried into this new chapter. "Take a punch, get back up," I repeated to myself, staring at the drill sergeant's boots, polished and stern. They were the gatekeepers to a world I was still learning to navigate, a world where my mettle would be tested, broken down, and ultimately rebuilt stronger. "Forward," I whispered, the word both command and promise as the cattle car hummed its way toward the unknown. With each passing second, my resolve grew, steeled by the knowledge that every trial was but a step toward becoming the man I was meant to be—resilient, hopeful, and ever moving forward.

The moment the cattle cars ground to a halt, a semblance of peace lingered, a deceptive calm before the storm. The barracks stood before us, relics of conflict past, their aging walls whispering tales of the countless feet that had trodden the same ground. As if on cue, the drill sergeants sprang into action with military precision, their calm exteriors giving way to a tempest of commands that shattered any illusions of gentleness. "Off the trucks, shit bags, let's go, move it!" Their voices thundered across the flat expanse, a cacophony that rattled my bones and spurred me into motion.

With the weight of my duffel bag digging into my shoulder, I stumbled off the cattle car, joining the sea of trainees shuffling toward our designated spots on the cement. "Put 'em down!" came the order, sharp as the snap of a flag in the wind. We complied, dropping our bags with a collective thud that seemed to echo off the barracks' stoic faces. But our efforts were met with scorn. "Too fucking slow, dirtbags! Pick 'em back up!" Each word stung like a slap, propelling my actions as I hoisted my bag once more, muscles protesting. "Hold 'em over your fat heads!" Sweat beaded on my brow as I thrust the heavy luggage upward, arms trembling under the strain. Around me, I could sense the collective tension, each of us silently praying not to be the first to falter. I felt the watchful eyes of the drill sergeants upon us, circling like vultures ready to swoop down on the vulnerable. My grip tightened, knuckles white, as I willed my arms to hold steady. It was in this crucible that we were being reshaped, our civilian selves stripped away layer by layer.

"Stay strong," I muttered to myself, an inner chant against the burn in my limbs. Resilience wasn't just physical; it was the flame of hope that flickered within, refusing to be snuffed out by adversity. I thought of Deb's unwavering belief in me, of Elaine's sacrifices, and Deb's battles. If they could endure life's harsh winds, I could withstand the gale of this moment. "Steady," I breathed, envisioning Sergeant Martinez's resolve, her strength a beacon. There was a lesson here, one of perseverance, camaraderie, and the unspoken bond forming between us all—each struggling figure a thread in the tapestry of fortitude. And somewhere beyond this trial lay the laughter of Greg, a reminder that luck was also our comrade-in-arms, often found in unexpected places.

In the shadow of these time-worn barracks, amid the cries of drill sergeants and the clatter of gear, I found an anchor in the storm—a vision of the man I was becoming. One forged in the fires of hardship yet buoyed by an undying optimism that whispered of victories yet to come. Muscles quivering, I hoisted my duffel bag above my head yet again, sweat beading on my forehead and dripping onto the dusty ground. The smell of earth mingled with the scent of exertion, filling the air as we all stood there, a collective of potential soldiers under the watchful gaze of our superiors.

"There's the weak link!" The shout cut through the heavy breathing around me, jolting my heart into a faster rhythm. A fellow recruit, his face red and contorted with effort, had succumbed to fatigue, his duffel bag crashing down beside him. The drill sergeants descended like vultures, their boots thudding ominously on the concrete. "DROP and give us twenty!" they commanded, their voices a unified bark of authority. The soldier's body hit the ground, arms trembling as he pushed against gravity, his efforts more a battle against his own limitations than a compliance with orders. "That's pathetic! EVERYONE DROP and give us twenty!" And so we complied, a symphony of thuds echoing as bodies met the ground. "Pick your bags up! Too slow! Put 'em back down!"

The chaos was a tangible thing, a beast that chewed on our resolve and spat out shards of broken morale. Glass shattered within bags; personal items became casualties of war before the real battle had even begun. "Pick 'em up! Put 'em down!" On and on it went until time lost meaning and all that remained were the commands and the relentless struggle to obey.

"So this is basic training," I gasped inwardly, each breath a labored conquest. Doubt gnawed at the edges of my conviction. "What the hell was I thinking?" The question was a weight, adding to the physical load I bore above me. Yet in that maelstrom of despair, a voice from within—or perhaps from a memory of a simpler time—whispered resilience into my ear. "It's about how hard you can get hit and keep moving forward. That's how winning is done." Rocky's gritty determination reverberated through the caverns of my mind. As the drill sergeants prowled between the ranks, seeking out the next victim of their orchestrated mayhem, I focused on that inner voice, allowing it to carry me through the tempest.

With a last herculean effort, I set the bag down gently, preserving what little remained inside. Eyes scanning the barracks for an unclaimed bunk, I felt the fibers of my being intertwining with those around me, each of us silently acknowledging the shared ordeal. We were no longer just individuals; we were becoming a unit—a concept larger than the sum of its parts. I claimed a bunk, its spartan simplicity a stark reminder of the journey ahead. As I lay there, allowing the ache in my limbs to ebb away, I realized that this was but the first of many tests. They would try to break us, but with each trial, we were being forged into something stronger.

"Resilience," I whispered to the quiet darkness, a promise to myself and an homage to those who believed in me. Tomorrow would bring new challenges, but tonight, I rested with the knowledge that hope was a stubborn flame and luck a companion ever waiting in the wings. Exhaustion had seeped into my bones, settling like sediment in a weary riverbed. I had fallen onto the bunk, an unforgiving slab of wood and thin mattress that now formed my nightly refuge. The green wool blanket scratched against my skin with every imperceptible movement, yet the sensation was lost to me, drowned beneath waves of fatigue that washed over my consciousness. Sleep, when it did claim me, was a merciful oblivion, one devoid of dreams or the relentless ache of muscles pushed beyond their limit.

In those precious hours of darkness, there was no basic training, no drill sergeants, no endless cycle of pushups and shouted commands. There was just the stillness of men too drained to even contemplate fear or failure. Yet as the adage goes, night is darkest just before dawn, and our dawn came heralded not by the gentle kiss of sunlight but by a cacophony that jolted us from slumber. The metallic clash of hammers hitting empty trash cans reverberated through the barracks, a symphony of chaos conducted by the very hands tasked with molding us into soldiers. We were on our feet before our minds could register the reason, instincts kicking in where thoughts lagged behind.

I scrambled upright, the unexpected brightness assaulting my eyes, amplifying the disorientation that clung to my mind like the last vestiges of sleep. My heart raced, and for a fleeting moment, I was back home in my bedroom, startled awake by a fierce storm. But the reality of my situation snapped into focus, the drill sergeants' silhouettes etched against the stark, artificial light, and the illusory comfort of home vanished like smoke.

"Move, move, move!" Their voices cut through the din, sharp and unyielding. There was no room for hesitation, no time to dwell on the soreness that protested with every hurried step. This was their domain, and we were merely players upon their stage, actors in a script written in the language of discipline and perseverance. As I fell into line, the echo of Rocky's words once again found its way to my inner sanctuary, a mantra amid the madness. "It ain't about how hard you hit. It's about how hard you can get hit and keep moving forward." It was this thread of hope, spun from the fabric of my own resolve, that I clung to—a lifeline in the maelstrom.

Luck, it seemed, had taken a back seat to the sheer will to survive, to adapt, to overcome. As the day's trials loomed ominously ahead, I held on to the notion that resilience was itself a form of good fortune. And if history had taught me anything, it was that even the longest and darkest nights eventually gave way to dawn. So with grit set in my jaw and determination fueling my spirit, I embraced the chaos. For in that moment, amid the hammering clangs and sergeants' cries, I understood that each challenge surmounted was another step toward the person I was meant to become.

The rhythm of military life settled into my bones, a relentless tempo that pushed me to the edge of my physical and mental limits. With each sunrise, the sergeants' relentless drills chiseled away at the remnants of who I had been, fashioning from the raw material of our collective resolve something harder, sharper. I quickly realized that success here was measured in silent obedience, in the uncomplaining acceptance of each new trial. Eyes forward, shoulders back, I became an embodiment of the discipline they demanded. The grueling exercises, the endless marches—all orchestrated to break us down, to strip away the individual and forge the soldier. It was a crucible, one that burned away the dross and left behind only the steel of our shared purpose.

Then came the day we were to face the gas chamber. Anxieties buzzed through the ranks like static as we donned our charcoal-lined suits and tightened our masks, sealing ourselves off from the world. Our breaths were audible in the claustrophobic silence, each inhale and exhale a testament to the tension that gripped us. We approached the gas chamber, an unassuming wooden structure that seemed far too mundane for the fear it inspired. But beneath its plain exterior lay a test of our trust in the equipment and in ourselves. Thirty souls filed in, a collective organism bound by trepidation and the will to overcome it.

As the door sealed shut behind us, I could feel my heart drumming against my chest, a staccato beat seeking reassurance in the midst of uncertainty. We stood shoulder to shoulder, a phalanx braced against an invisible enemy, and within that small hut, we found solidarity. There was comfort in knowing that we were not alone in our fear, that each of us bore the weight of this moment together.

"Steady," I whispered to myself, the words a lifeline cast into the roiling sea of my thoughts. "Steady." In this place, where every breath was an act of faith, hope became the armor that shielded us from our doubts. And so with lungs burning and eyes watering, we proved to ourselves that we could stand firm, even when the very air we breathed was turned against us. The deceptive calm within the gas chamber was a stark contrast to the chaos of our training outside. Cocooned in my full suit and mask, I stood shoulder-to-shoulder with my fellow trainees, surrounded by the dull wood of the hut's interior. The glass block windows filtered the harsh sunlight into less intimidating beams that danced across the space. There wasn't a hint of danger in the air—no stench, no acrid taste on the tongue, no burning sensation in the lungs. For a fleeting moment, it felt like just another drill, another box to check off in the endless list of tasks that formed our basic training.

"Remove your gloves," came the order, shattering the illusion of safety. I obeyed, peeling the protective fabric from my hands. It was as if I had plunged them straight into a fire. The sting was sudden, vicious, an invisible blaze scorching my skin. A collective gasp rose from the trainees; we all felt it, the raw intensity of pain that cut through our drilled-in stoicism. Our hands were on fire, and there was nothing but air to blame. "Remove your masks," the drill sergeants commanded next. My heart hammered against my ribcage.

If this is what my hands feel like, what unimaginable agony awaits my face? But hesitation was not an option. With trembling fingers, I reached up and unsealed the mask from my head, holding my breath as if it might somehow shield me from the inevitable onslaught. As the mask slid off, a searing heat lashed at my face. My eyes watered, and I bit back a curse. We stood exposed, vulnerable to the riot control gas that we now knew was very much present, even though it remained an unseen enemy.

"Sound off! Your ABCs, name, rank, serial number, chain of command!" bellowed the drill sergeants. We could barely breathe, much less recite what they ordered us to. It was more than an exercise; it was a testament to our ability to function under duress, to maintain composure when every instinct screamed otherwise. Clarity of thought amid the fog of discomfort became our immediate struggle. My voice joined the cacophony of others, each of us desperately clinging to the familiar sequence of letters, the identity we'd been assigned, the structure of command that tethered us to order amid the turmoil. This was resilience in its purest form. Not the absence of pain or fear but the will to stand firm in their presence. As the biting chemicals ravaged my senses, I found a sliver of hope within the torment. Each second endured was a small victory, a silent declaration that I was still here, still fighting, still becoming the soldier I vowed to be.

"Adapt and overcome." The mantra was a lifeline now, pulled taut by the gravity of the moment. My past, rife with its own trials and tribulations, seemed to echo around me, reminding me that I had weathered storms before. This, too, would pass, and I would emerge stronger for it. In the relentless pursuit of progress, luck played no part—it was the steadfast belief in one's own capacity to push forward, to rise above, and to transform hardship into hope. And as the drill sergeants watched us wrangle with the gas, I understood that this struggle was not meant to break us. It was here to show us the depths of our own tenacity—and in those depths, I found an unwavering light that would guide me through whatever darkness lay ahead. The acrid stench of the gas filled my nostrils, a pungent reminder of the ordeal's reality. My body revolted against the invisible assailant as snot streamed unchecked, cascading to the concrete floor in rivulets of shared misery. Around me, fellow trainees succumbed to their own battles—stomachs churning, contents expelled in an involuntary act of defiance against the searing air that enveloped us.

Through tear-blurred eyes, I witnessed a spectacle of desperation: one soldier from Kentucky, his frame silhouetted against the dim light filtering through the hut's windows, charged headlong toward the wall. A futile attempt to escape the engulfing torment. His impact with the unyielding surface was met with a hollow thud—a stark testament to the futility of resistance in the face of such overwhelming adversity. Laughter, cruel and biting, cut through the cacophony of coughs and retches. The drill sergeants found humor in our suffering, their mirth incongruous amid the chaos. They stood firm, their authority unshaken by the scene before them, as they demanded we articulate the words that tethered us to order amid the turmoil.

And there it was again, that indomitable spirit echoing within me—the voice of Rocky Balboa, a cinematic hero who had become an unwitting mentor through the years. "The world ain't all sunshine and rainbows, it's a very mean and nasty place."

The words resonated deeply, a mantra for survival amid the trials unfolding around me. I nodded to myself—a subtle acknowledgment of the truth in those words—as I stumbled out of the hut, each step a triumph over the malevolent haze that sought to claim my resolve. Within the haze, within the laughter of drill sergeants and the cries of my comrades, there was a lesson being etched into my very soul.

Emerging from the wooden hut, gasping for air and grappling with the sting of the gas on my skin, I found solace in the crisp, outside air. The sun's rays were a gentle hand compared to the chaos within. We lined up as instructed, our hands awkwardly hovering by our sides. The drill sergeants' eyes roamed over us, searching for any sign of defiance. One of my squad mates, a usually disciplined guy with sweat still glistening on his brow, made a beeline for the porta potty, against the instructions given to us just a short time ago. Our sergeant, a silent shadow, trailed him without uttering a word.

The moment the door clanked shut, the drill sergeant's prediction unfurled into reality. A scream tore through the morning calm, a raw, visceral sound that spoke volumes of the agony he must have been feeling. "This is what happens when you don't fucking listen to us, you ignorant maggots!" the drill sergeant barked. The rest of us winced, a stark reminder that every action here had weight, consequences that could not be outrun.

As night fell on the barracks, so did an unexpected chill within me. I coughed through the darkness, a relentless echo that filled the space between the creaking bunks. My body was rebelling, and there was no silencing its outcry. It was clear; I was allergic to one or more of the chemicals that lingered in my lungs. My fellow soldiers tossed and turned, their irritation palpable. But beneath their frustration, I sensed a tinge of concern—after all, we were in this together.

Dawn broke with a new challenge; a ruck march heavier than the bags we carried. It was another test of endurance, a crucible designed to forge us into something greater. As we trudged over the miles, my chest tightened, each breath a labor. Yet amid the physical strain, my spirit remained unyielding. For each step was a step toward becoming the soldier I aspired to be—trained in hand-to-hand combat, proficient with grenades, adept at the machine gun.

The journey was long, and the path uncertain, but I was learning that the essence of hope lies not in the absence of adversity but in the persistence through it. In these formative moments, as much as my body ached to surrender, I held on to the belief that luck favors those who dare to endure. This was the battlefield of self-transformation, and I was determined to emerge victorious, no matter the personal cost. "Adapt and overcome." This mantra wasn't just words— it was my lifeline, my pledge, my unwavering commitment to rise above the trials and seize the promise of a new day.

With each step, the weight of my gear melded with the heaviness in my chest, a leaden reminder of the invisible battle raging within me. The ruck march was relentless—a torturous pilgrimage across unforgiving terrain, meant to temper our spirits and bodies alike. But as my breaths grew shallow and sharp, I could feel the grip of pneumonia tightening like an unyielding vice. "Keep it up, keep moving!" barked the drill sergeant, his voice a jagged edge cutting through the haze of pain and fatigue. Yet even as his words lashed at me, Rocky's enduring mantra reverberated in my mind: *It's not about how hard you can hit, it's about how hard you can* get *hit and keep moving forward...*

I endeavored to embody those words, to push beyond the threshold of endurance. Each footfall was a testament to will, to the indefatigable human spirit that refuses to succumb. But despite my mental fortitude, the body has its limits, and mine were rapidly approaching. The world began to spin, a carousel of blurred greens and browns, and I felt my knees buckle. The ground came up to meet me, and all at once, the sergeant's shouts faded into a distant echo. As I lay there, the foliage canopy overhead spinning, I sensed the change in him. The hard lines of his face softened momentarily, replaced by something resembling fear—perhaps even respect—as he radioed for help.

Time lost meaning as I convalesced in the sterile confines of the hospital, the rhythmic beeps of machines syncing with my own fragile breaths. Two weeks of white walls and whispered reassurances from nurses who became temporary guardians in this unexpected detour on my journey. Upon my return to training, the landscape had shifted; familiar faces were absent, replaced by those of strangers. They were a cohort untouched by the trials I'd faced, standing on the precipice of their own encounter with the gas chamber. Dread settled heavily upon me, a cloak woven from memories of agony and the sting of betrayal by my own body. With a doctor's note clutched in my hand—a shield crafted from medical authority—I approached Sergeant Martinez. Her presence was a beacon amid the uncertainty, her reputation for fairness preceding her like a whispered promise.

"Sergeant," I began, the paper trembling in my grasp, "I've got orders here from the doc. No gas chamber for me. Severe allergic reaction." Though I braced for dismissal or disdain, I saw neither in her eyes. Instead, there was an almost imperceptible nod, a silent acknowledgment of the battle scars I bore, both visible and veiled. She took the note, reading the colonel's scrawl, and I held my breath, waiting for the verdict that would seal my fate.

"Understood," she said simply, handing back the note. And in that moment, I felt the tightness in my chest ease—not from the relief of cleared lungs but from the weight of worry lifting. That day,

I learned a new kind of resilience—one that didn't merely involve enduring physical trials but also navigating the unpredictable currents of circumstance. It was a lesson in hope, a realization that sometimes luck doesn't just happen; it's granted by those rare individuals who see beyond the uniform to the person beneath.

And so with renewed determination, I stepped back into the rhythm of training, a solitary figure amongst a sea of camouflage, marching toward an uncertain future with unwavering resolve. The morning was crisp, the kind that bites at your lungs—a reminder that despite my recent brush with illness, I was alive. The unforgiving concrete beneath my boots felt like a testament to my resolve as I walked toward the drill sergeant, the doctor's note a flimsy shield in my hand. "Here, Sergeant," I said, offering up the paper with a mix of defiance and trepidation, its edges damp with the sweat of my palm.

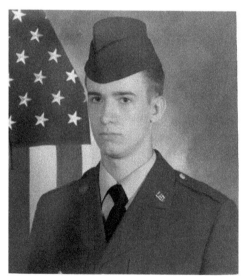

If I look angry here, it's because I am. This was taken after I recovered from pneumonia for the second time in basic training.

He snatched it from me, his eyes not meeting mine as he read the colonel's orders. For a fleeting moment, there was silence, a pause in the cacophony of military life. And then the world narrowed to the sound of tearing paper. "What is this, SHIT BAG?" His voice shattered any illusion of understanding. The crumpled pieces of the note fell to the ground, a discarded plea. "Gear up! You're going in first!"

My heart hammered against my rib cage, a drumbeat of impending doom. Even as I donned the chemical suit, my mind screamed in protest. I had survived the merciless embrace of pneumonia only to be thrust back into its jaws. "Move it, move it!"

They herded us toward the chamber, a small wooden building that stood as a silent judge, indifferent to my predicament. Each step felt like a betrayal of my body's recent memory of hospital sheets and whispered conversations by my bedside. "Mask on!" the order came, and we complied, sealing ourselves off from the world. Yet even behind the mask, I could taste the dread, thick and bitter.

"Enter!" they commanded, and we did. One by one, we stepped into the hut, our sanctuary from the gas turned prison.

"Remove your masks!"

The world spun, reality blurring at the edges as I struggled to obey, each breath a fiery agony. My lungs screamed, my vision clouded with tears—not from the gas but from the pain, the utter helplessness of being ignored, forced into harm's way. It wasn't long before the symptoms clawed their way back, racking my body with coughs, each one a brutal reminder of the fragility of my health and the fierce will to survive that refused to be extinguished.

"Clear out!" The drill sergeant's laughter echoed as we spilled from the chamber, a chaotic mess of human suffering. "Stand down, soldier," one of them barked as I doubled over, gasping for air that would not come. But my battle was far from over. The colonel arrived, his fury palpable. He stormed through the infirmary, his words a torrent as he demanded the commander on the phone. I watched, through a haze of oxygen masks and IV drips, as the consequences unfolded. The drill sergeant who had been so quick to dismiss my condition was stripped of his rank, his contempt for my well-being sealing his fate.

As I lay there, recovering for the second time, the echo of Rocky's wisdom filled the sterile space—"It's about how hard you can get hit and keep moving forward." It became a mantra, the rhythm to which I set the pace of my recovery.

Discouraged and feeling defeated, I picked up the phone and called my mother. She listened patiently as I poured out my frustration and anger, the weight of my experiences weighing heavily on my shoulders. "I don't know if I can do this, Mom," I confessed, my voice trembling with emotion. "I feel like giving up." There was a long pause as if she was choosing her words carefully.

Finally, she spoke. "Quitting is always an option," she said softly. "But remember, if you quit now, you might be a quitter for the rest of your life."

Her words hit me like a punch to the gut. I had never thought of myself as a quitter before. In fact, I prided myself on my determination and perseverance. "But it's so hard," I protested weakly.

"I know it's hard," she replied with sympathy in her voice. "But nothing worth having comes easy."

Her words struck a chord within me. She was right. This wasn't going to be easy, but it was something that I wanted more than anything else. "You're strong, honey," she continued. "You've been through so much already and you've come out on top every time. Don't let this defeat you."

Tears welled up in my eyes as her words filled me with renewed determination and courage. My mother had always been my biggest supporter and cheerleader, even from hundreds of miles away. "I won't give up," I promised her.

"That's my man," she said proudly. "I believe in you."

We talked for a little while longer before saying our goodbyes. As I hung up the phone, I felt a newfound strength coursing through me. My mother's encouragement had given me the boost I needed to keep moving forward.

I clung to the hope that sprang forth in those moments, the belief that resilience was more than just physical—it was the courage to face adversity head-on, to find allies in unexpected places, and to recognize that every setback was a setup for a comeback. There was luck in survival, yes, but there was also the unwavering spirit that refused to yield, to bend, to break.

And so amid the clatter of trays and the whispers of nurses, I plotted my return to the ranks, to the relentless march of those who wore the uniform, knowing that whatever lay ahead, I was equipped not just with armor and arms but with an unshakable resolve and the quiet conviction that sometimes, the hardest battles were fought within the chambers of the heart. Emerging from the fog of illness and the shadow of my last encounter with authority, I found myself back in the fray, the cadence of marching boots a familiar anthem to my ears.

Basic training resumed its relentless pace around me, but this time with a marked difference—I carried within me not just the weight of my pack but the weight of experience, the knowledge that resilience was as crucial to survival as the air I breathed.

The days blurred into one another, each sunrise bringing new challenges, each sunset seeing them conquered. As I pushed through the physical demands and mental rigor, a newfound determination settled in my bones. I was not just enduring; I was excelling. When the final test scores were placed in my hands, the numbers nearly leapt off the page. A near-perfect score stared back at me, confirming what I had only begun to suspect—I had more potential than I ever gave myself credit for. The army saw it, too, informing me that every job was within reach, a smorgasbord of opportunity laid out before me. Yet amid the myriad paths I could take, my gaze fixed upon communications and electronics. There was something about the intricacies of circuits and signals that resonated with me, a silent language that spoke of connection and understanding.

The weeks at Fort Gordon, Georgia, were a whirlwind of learning and growth. With each lesson on transmitters and receivers, I pieced together not just machines but fragments of my future. The training was rigorous and challenging, but I met it head-on, the words of encouragement from my instructors fueling my resolve. A brief respite at home served as a reminder of how far I'd come. My family's eyes mirrored the pride I felt swelling within me, their support an unspoken promise that no matter where my journey took me, I would never truly be alone. Those 180 days passed like a dream, a life once so familiar now tinged with the promise of change.

Then, standing on the precipice of the unknown, I boarded a plane to Germany. The year was 1983, and Bobby Quayle, at the tender age of seventeen, was wide-eyed and green, yet beneath that youthful exterior beat the heart of someone who had faced down demons and emerged victorious. As the aircraft lifted into the sky, I couldn't help but look down at the shrinking landscape below, each passing cloud a testament to the unpredictable nature of life. What awaited me in Germany? I couldn't say for certain, but the anticipation of discovery filled my chest with a buoyant hope.

In those moments, suspended between earth and sky, I realized that life is less about the destination and more about the journey. It's not the accolades or achievements that define us but the grit and grace with which we pursue our dreams. It's about rising after every fall, about the quiet courage that whispers, "Keep going" when everything else screams for surrender. And so as I crossed the threshold into a new chapter, it was with the knowledge that I was not merely moving toward something great—I was already living it. This was my odyssey, a tapestry woven from threads of hardship and triumph, and I was ready to see where the pattern would lead.

CHAPTER 6

EUROPEAN ADVENTURE

The thrum of the C-130's engines was a constant companion, vibrating through my bones as I settled into my jump seat, surrounded by the olive drab interior of the military transport. My fellow soldiers, some fresh-faced like me, others with lines of experience etched into their features, were a tapestry of anticipation and weariness. We were an airborne mosaic of America's bravest—some cradling photographs of loved ones, while others whispered reassurances to children too young to understand the journey. I gripped the cold metal beneath me, allowing a mixture of fear and excitement to course through me. This was it—the leap into the unknown that would test my resolve and shape my destiny.

The unfamiliar weight of my issued gear served as a reminder of the responsibility I had shouldered. It was a tangible expression of my commitment—a promise to serve and protect, even in a land whose tongue I could not speak, whose culture was a mystery waiting to be unraveled.

As the plane lumbered through the skies toward Germany, I closed my eyes against the noise, seeking solace in the quiet spaces of my mind. There, I replayed the conversation with the elderly man at the airport—the one who had unwittingly become a mentor in those brief moments before boarding. His presence had been unassuming, yet something about him commanded respect. He had shared his wisdom generously, speaking with the authority of someone who had lived a thousand lifetimes in one. His advice, though imparted quickly, had taken root in my heart. It was a seed of guidance, planted deep within the fertile soil of youthful optimism and naivety.

"Embrace the journey," he had said, his voice somehow both commanding and gentle. "Let this new world be your teacher, and you its willing student."

Even amid the cacophony of the aircraft's cavernous belly, I clung to his words. They were a mantra, a beacon to guide me through the maze of challenges and opportunities that lay ahead. Every mile that separated me from home was another step toward becoming the man I aspired to be—one molded by trials, tenacity, and the courage to embrace the unforeseen.

I pondered the path that had led me here, a boy from a small town now soaring over international waters, bound for a duty station steeped in history and tradition. The gravity of what I was undertaking began to settle upon me, but rather than weighing me down, it became the wings upon which my aspirations took flight. "Germany," I whispered to myself, tasting the word, letting it symbolize all the adventures to come. With each passing second, the country was drawing nearer, and with it the promise of transformation. I was no longer the person who had boarded this plane; I was becoming someone new, shaped by the hands of fate and the choices I was yet to make.

One thing was certain: I would remember the colonel's parting words and cherish the serendipitous encounter that had provided them. In the symphony of life's uncertainties, his voice would be a recurring note, harmonizing with my own burgeoning story of resilience and hope. The bustle of the airport had faded into a murmur as I sat, lost in thought, awaiting my flight to Bamberg. My gaze lingered on the tarmac, where planes taxied with purposeful grace, steel birds on an endless journey. The anticipation of my new life ahead mingled with trepidation, a silent storm brewing within me. I sat back, taking in the hum of the airport around me, feeling strangely solitary yet connected to an expansive future. Each footstep toward the boarding gate carried the weight of purpose, each heartbeat a drumroll to the adventure that awaited. This was no longer just an assignment or a stint abroad; it was a proving ground for my character, a canvas upon which my story would unfold in vibrant strokes of courage and curiosity.

He materialized beside me without fanfare, an unassuming figure whose presence gently nudged at the edges of my awareness. When he greeted me, his voice carried a familiar timbre that resonated oddly within my memory. His features were etched with stories untold, and though we had never met, something about him seemed like a reflection from a past life. "Hello, young man," the stranger said, his eyes crinkling with warmth. He extended his hand, weathered yet strong. "Retired Colonel. Heading to Germany too. Space-A," he added, explaining the privilege of travel offered to those who have served. His words fell like breadcrumbs on the path I was about to tread, hints of wisdom waiting to be gathered.

As the conversation unfolded, his question about my destination hung in the air between us. "Bamberg," I replied, the name of the town rolling off my tongue with uncertainty. "I'm… It's all so new to me."

His hand came to rest on my shoulder, a comforting weight that grounded me to the moment. "Listen closely," he began, his tone imbued with the kind of gravity that demanded attention. "Germany is going to be an adventure, and you, my friend, are at its threshold." His eyes held mine, their depths twinkling with the knowledge of countless experiences. "Embrace it. Learn from it."

The colonel's voice was a calm baritone as he painted the picture of life in Germany and two distinct groups of soldiers there, that second group—their nights marred by anger and regret—confined within the close quarters of local dive bars. "They rarely leave the base," he said, his gaze unwavering, "and when they do, their experiences… Well, let's just say they're far from what you'd want." He told me how those soldiers would swell the ranks of dimly lit establishments where the odds were stacked against any kind of meaningful connection. I could almost see it, the frustration boiling over into brawls, the walk back to the barracks under a sky devoid of stars, spirits as clouded as the German beers that fueled them.

"Thank you, sir," I said earnestly, a sense of relief washing over me. To know that such unhappiness was a choice rather than a fate gave me a newfound confidence. It was a trap I could sidestep, a path I didn't have to tread. I leaned in, eager for any further wisdom he might share. He straightened up, his eyes locking onto mine with an intensity that rooted me to the spot.

"One more thing," he began, his voice dropping to an almost conspiratorial hush. "If you are ever asked to perform any mission, no matter how difficult the task may seem at the time, you respond with 'Yes, sir' and perform that mission to the best of your ability."

The weight of his words felt like a sacred charge, a commandment I would carry with me through every trial ahead. "Understood, sir," I replied, my chest swelling with a mix of pride and trepidation. This wasn't just advice; it was a directive for life, a key to unlock honor in the shadow of challenge.

As he rose to board his flight, he turned back to me, a cryptic note in his voice. "You have a lot of important things to do over there," he said, leaving the sentence hanging in the air like a question without an answer.

"Sir, what do you mean by 'important things'?" I called after him, but he had already blended into the crowd. I scanned the bustling terminal, searching for the familiar figure, but he had vanished as if he were a ghost or a figment conjured by my anxious mind. Left with the echo of his counsel, I felt a strange kinship with this man whose name I couldn't recall. His words clung to me, burrowed deep into my thoughts. They were a compass, guiding me not only toward embracing a foreign land but also toward embracing the essence of who I wanted to become—a man defined by resilience and an unwavering commitment to face whatever lay ahead.

In that instant, surrounded by the hustle of travelers and the cacophony of departure announcements, I felt a kinship with this man. A mentor had appeared when I needed one most, offering a compass for the journey ahead. Though his next words have since been lost to time, the essence of his advice remained, a beacon to guide me through the labyrinth of the unknown. As he departed, leaving me with his parting wisdom, I sensed the magnitude of the opportunity before me. I was a soldier, yes, but also a seeker of horizons, a gatherer of experiences. The retired colonel's counsel would be the undercurrent to my actions, shaping the choices that lay ahead.

"Germany," I breathed once more, feeling the word settle into my bones. It was no longer just a place but a promise—a canvas upon which my story would unfold. There, amid the echoes of history and the whispers of destiny, I would find my footing. With every step, I would carve out a space of my own, becoming a testament to resilience, hope, and perhaps a little luck. The retired colonel's hand had weighed on my shoulder like an anchor, steadying the tumult of apprehensions swirling through my mind. I could feel the thrumming energy of the aircraft, its pulse syncing with the racing beat of my heart. This was it—the threshold of a new chapter, and his words were the prelude to what my life would become.

"Two distinct groups of soldiers," he had said, his voice etched with the gravitas of experience. And as the plane lifted off, soaring into the boundless sky, I felt myself being torn between two potential fates. The thought of being among those who loathed their time in Germany chilled me. I wasn't just another recruit; I was Bobby Quayle, seeker of silver linings, a man who'd learned to dance in the rain rather than wait for the storm to pass.

I peered out the small window, catching glimpses of the world shrinking below, and imagined the soldiers who had taken this very flight before me. Which group had they fallen into? What choices had they made that I could learn from?

"Get away from the base," the colonel's advice echoed in my mind, reverberating with every hum of the engine. A simple strategy yet profound. To love Germany, one must embrace it—its language, its culture, its people. It was about stepping beyond the shadow of the base, where misunderstandings festered, and finding the places where light shone on American soldiers with warmth and welcome.

My reflection stared back at me from the oval glass, eyes filled with hopeful determination. I would be part of the first group, not because of luck but because I would make it so. I'd muster the courage to venture into the unfamiliar, to bridge divides with broken German if need be. I would seek out the Germany that lay beyond the reach of rumors and resentments, where camaraderie waited in unassuming guesthouses and quaint village squares.

In that moment, strapped into my seat amid fellow soldiers and their families, the path forward seemed clear. Upon touching German soil, I would lay down roots not through force but through understanding. The seeds of friendship and respect would be planted with each handshake, each halting phrase in a new tongue, each shared laugh echoing through cobblestone streets.

"Embrace it. Learn from it," the colonel's parting words resounded within me. And as the plane charted its course over oceans and continents, I charted my own. With a notebook resting on my knee, I began jotting down phrases, landmarks, customs—anything and everything that might aid my journey.

Germany loomed on the horizon, not as a challenge to be endured but as an adventure to be cherished. I would not simply occupy space there; I would thrive, turning strangers into friends, foreign streets into familiar pathways, and uncertainty into stories worth telling.

And when doubt whispered its insidious song, I would remember the colonel's wisdom, the promise in his eyes that spoke of hidden fortunes waiting for those bold enough to claim them. Yes, I would be among those who loved Germany and, in doing so, might just learn to love a new facet of myself.

As I settled into my seat on the aircraft, the outside world shrank away, leaving me with my reflections and the boundless skies. The colonel's parting words lingered, a beacon of hope and a reminder that I was master of my fate, able to steer my course through uncharted territories with determination and grit. Whatever "important things" awaited, I was ready to meet them with a resolute "Yes, sir" and a heart full of hope.

The hum of the C-130's engines was a steady drone, like a persistent whisper of the journey ahead. As the aircraft descended, I pressed my face against the cool windowpane, gazing at the patchwork of green fields and clusters of buildings below. The German countryside sprawled out like a canvas of history and modernity intertwined, with old stone houses huddling alongside sleek industrial structures. My pulse quickened; this was a land pulsing with stories, and soon, I would be part of its narrative.

"Landing in Frankfurt," the pilot's voice crackled over the intercom, signaling our imminent arrival. My heart skipped. I was on the precipice of the unknown, yet I couldn't help but feel a surge of hope. This was my moment to seize, to venture beyond the confines of familiarity and into the embrace of a new culture. I was determined to belong to the group that reveled in the richness of this place.

I disembarked, shouldering my life packed into two duffel bags, each step a march into my future. The military bus rumbled toward the barracks, a solemn carrier delivering fresh faces to their fates. As it halted, I stepped onto German soil for the first time, a tangible transition that solidified my resolve.

Approaching the barracks, I was struck by the starkness of the building—its stoic facade a testament to the countless boots that had tread its halls. Suddenly, a window thrust open above, shattering my introspection. "NEW BOOT! NEW BOOT!" a voice boomed, the words piercing through the crisp air, pointing an invisible finger squarely at me.

Heads turned, laughter erupted, and the chant spread like wildfire. "NEW BOOT! NEW BOOT, LAME RECRUIT!" The sing-song taunt cascaded from one window to the next, a chorus of jests from faces I had yet to know. But instead of wilting under their mockery, something within me stirred—a fire kindled by challenge.

This was no different than any other hurdle I'd encountered in life: the skepticism when I enlisted, the doubt that shadowed my every ambition. Yet here I was, standing firm on foreign ground, ready to prove my mettle. Their words were not shackles but a gauntlet thrown at my feet, an invitation to rise.

"Welcome to Germany," I muttered to myself, a wry smile tugging at the corners of my mouth. With squared shoulders and a spirit undeterred, I marched toward the barracks door. The teasing faded into the background, drowned out by the drumbeat of my own determination. I was not just another "new boot" lost in the shuffle—I was Bobby Quayle, and I was going to make this place my home.

And somewhere, perhaps watching from a distance or merely a presence felt in spirit, I sensed the old colonel nodding in approval. I carried his wisdom with me, etched into my resolve. For I knew that the path to love and embrace this country lay in my own hands, and I was ready to grasp it with both.

The weight of the duffel bags hit the ground with a thud, echoing my defiance. My voice cut through the jeers like a knife. "WHO THE FUCK ARE YOU CALLING LAME!" Their laughter stung, but it didn't deter me. I hoisted one bag onto my back, its contents pressing heavily against me—sixty pounds of life I was carrying into this new chapter.

"OH YEAH? Can a lame recruit do this?" The challenge had left my lips before I could second-guess myself. Dropping to the ground, I started pumping out push-ups, each one a silent testament to my determination.

"HA! Look at the BOOT, he's trying to be hardcore!" their mockery rang out.

Another voice joined in, counting mockingly, "One, one, one, one..." as though my efforts were meaningless.

I gritted my teeth, feeling the burn intensify with every descent and ascent. Ten push-ups passed, then twenty, the numbers stacking up as my arms shook with the effort. Thirty, forty. By the time I reached fifty, a hush had descended over the onlookers. Standing back up, my arms trembled with exertion, but my resolve was ironclad. "How many of you LAME asses can do what I just did?"

Their silence was my answer. I strode toward the barracks entrance, a bold grin plastered across my face, my heart pounding with triumph. This display wasn't merely about strength or stamina; it was my declaration of presence, my refusal to be reduced to the label of "new boot" without a fight.

As the door swung open, I stepped inside, leaving behind the echoes of their taunts and the sensation of victory warming my chest. Inside these walls would be countless challenges but also opportunities—opportunities to learn, to grow, and to show what I was truly made of.

In that moment, I felt an understanding, a kinship with every person who ever dared to prove themselves in the face of adversity. With each step forward, I carried with me the spirit of resilience that had been forged through every trial I'd faced—each struggle a steppingstone leading me here.

The old colonel's words played in my mind like a mantra, reminding me that my journey in Germany was one of discovery and engagement. I was not here to simply exist within the confines of the base; I was here to embrace the culture, the people, the very essence of this place. And I was ready to take that leap, to find joy in the unknown.

"Welcome home, Bobby," I whispered to myself, feeling the weight of my duffel bags now not as a burden but as a promise of the life I was about to build. A life filled with hope, reinforced by the knowledge that every challenge surmounted only added to the story I was writing with each breath I took.

It was early Saturday morning and the chill of the German morning seeped into the barracks, and I pulled my green army-issue blanket a little tighter around me. From my bunk, I watched as the pale light of dawn began to snake its way across the floor, illuminating the spartan simplicity of the room I now called home. The first stirring murmurs of my roommates punctuated the quiet as they too began to wake, their shadows stretching long against the wall like silent giants from tales of old.

"What are you going to do this weekend, boot?"

The question snapped me back to reality, and I turned to see one of my roommates eyeing me with a mix of curiosity and playful taunting. I straightened up on the bunk, rolling my shoulders to shake off the stiffness from a night on the unforgiving mattress. "This 'boot' is going to start his weekend by putting a boot in your ass if you keep calling me THAT!" I shot back, more out of habit than actual irritation. A round of laughter erupted from the others, the sound bouncing off the cinder block walls and filling the room with a sense of camaraderie that was hard to resist.

"Ease up, man," he chuckled, shaking his head. "We're just messing with you. But seriously, we're heading out tonight. Gonna show you what town's got to offer. You in?"

The invitation hung in the air, tempting. I could already picture the neon glow of bar signs, the clinking of glasses, the easy forgetfulness that came with a night of revelry. But behind that image loomed the colonel's advice, a beacon reminding me there was more to discover beyond the haze of alcohol and the same old stories retold in dimly lit corners.

"Thanks, but I haven't decided yet," I said, my voice steady despite the uncertainty that fluttered in my chest. Their plans, though not without appeal, felt like an echo of something I was meant to leave behind. I was here for growth, for experience, for life—and that life wasn't going to find me if I stayed within the comfortable bubble of familiarity.

"Suit yourself, boot." Another roommate shrugged, already moving on to other topics as they planned their evening.

I leaned back, letting the moment wash over me—the excitement of my peers, the anticipation of the unknown, the pulse of a new world just beyond the barracks' walls. I thought about the colonel again, his eyes earnest and knowing as he imparted wisdom that felt ages old yet undeniably relevant. "Two groups of soldiers," his voice echoed in my mind, a guiding light in the uncertainty.

As the chatter around me faded into white noise, my heart made the decision before my mind could catch up. It was settled—I would carve my own path, explore Germany with fresh eyes, and embrace whatever adventures awaited me. It was time to step out of the shadow of expectations and into the sunlight of possibility. *Introspection* was the word that came to mind as I finally rose from my bed, determination settling into my bones. This weekend marked the beginning of something—of many things, perhaps. And I would meet it head-on, armed with hope, resilience, and a dash of luck that seemed to follow those who dared to chase their dreams.

With a determined exhale, I hoisted my duffel bag onto the bed and began to pack. The weight of decision pressed against me, but it was a good weight, one that felt like purpose being loaded into my very fibers. The colonel's advice rang true, and I could almost hear the timbre of his voice guiding me.

"There are two groups of soldiers in Germany," he had said, and I knew, without a shard of doubt, which group I intended to belong to.

"Going to go explore Germany a little bit!" I announced to the room, my words slicing through their plans like a knife through soft butter. The seasoned cadence of my voice surprised me, a stark contrast to the idle banter around me. My roommates paused, casting curious glances my way as they absorbed my sudden declaration.

I zipped up my bag, feeling the fabric strain against the promise of adventure. It was a four-day weekend ahead, the first taste of freedom in this new land, and my paycheck lay snug in my pocket—a paper-bound comrade ready for duty. *Let's have some fun*, I thought, the phrase imbued with more than just lightheartedness; it was a rallying cry for the life I'd yet to discover. As I shouldered my bag and stepped out of the barracks, I felt the eyes of my roommates on my back. Their laughter and jeers did not follow me; instead, there was only silence, a respectful acknowledgment of the path I chose to tread.

The air outside was crisp, carrying whispers of history and secrets of the cobblestone streets that wound between buildings like veins. I took a deep breath, letting the foreign scents fill my lungs, and with each step, I felt the chains of trepidation fall away. A sense of hope unfurled within me, bright and stubborn as the sun peeking through overcast skies. My journey would take me beyond the gates, past the looming shadows of expectations, and into the golden fields of opportunity that stretched out before me. Each footfall was a word in the story I was beginning to write—resilience etched in the gravel, hope in the horizon, and luck, perhaps, waiting around the next bend.

That pivotal decision to venture forth on my own was the turning point I hadn't known I needed. It led me down roads less traveled, where friendships blossomed like wildflowers along the path. The colonel had been right. This wasn't just about finding joy in a foreign country; it was about discovering the strength within myself to seek out that joy, to grasp it tightly and let it propel me forward. With every mile I traversed, every smile from a stranger, every word of broken German that fell from my lips, I wove a tapestry of experiences that would color my narrative for years to come. I was no longer just a soldier on foreign soil; I was an explorer in a land that promised growth, connection, and the kind of camaraderie that transcends borders. And as the weekend unfolded into memories I'd carry forever, I realized the truth embedded in the colonel's wisdom: our lives are defined not by the places we're stationed but by the steps we dare to take beyond them.

The weight of my duffel bags seemed lighter somehow as I crossed the sprawling base, buoyed by a sense of adventure and the echo of that wise, old colonel's advice. The gravel crunched under my boots, each step marking my progress toward an unknown yet thrilling future. The air was crisp, filled with the scent of freedom and diesel; it was the aroma of possibility.

"Taxi!" My voice sounded strange, tinged with an accent of excitement and a sliver of trepidation. A yellow Mercedes-Benz cab pulled up to the curb, its emblem a beacon of unexpected luxury in this utilitarian world I had come to know. "*Bahnhof bitte*," I managed to articulate in my most confident broken German, pointing to the train station on a crumpled map.

"*Ja wohl!*" the driver's affirmation came back like a promise, his words ringing with the warmth of welcome. Billy Joel played on the radio as we drove away from the familiarity of the base, the military structures dwindled in the rearview mirror replaced by the sprawling German countryside. The houses were neat, precise, and there was an order to the chaos of nature here that felt both foreign and inviting.

At the train station, I stood before the ticket window, dwarfed by the timetables and maps adorning the walls. The colonel's voice replayed in my mind, a guiding mantra urging me to venture beyond the expected. "Get away from the base and the nearest city, and the Germans will treat you like a king." With audacity as my compass, I closed my eyes and let fate take the wheel. My finger danced across the timetable, a ballet of chance, before coming to rest on a name that felt as random as any: Roedental. Destiny, it seemed, had a sense of humor.

"*Roedental, hin und zurück bitte,*" I said, fumbling over the syllables but proud of my attempt, nonetheless.

The cashier nodded, punching the details into her machine with mechanical precision. I couldn't help but wonder if she knew how momentous this small transaction was for me—a ticket to a new chapter, a passageway to self-discovery. As I sat, waiting for the train, I watched people bustling about, each lost in their own stories. Their faces were canvases of routine, etched with the lines of everyday concerns, and yet here I was, a mere teenager of just seventeen years, embarking on an odyssey that would define the very fabric of my being. The train's arrival broke my reverie with a metallic symphony of screeches and hisses. It was time.

Stepping aboard, I felt the finality of the act. This train ride wasn't just about distance; it was about bridging the gap between who I was and who I could become. The journey ahead was mine alone, a path paved with resilience and hope. Somewhere along those steel tracks lay a friendship that would change my life, a bond forged in the fires of shared experiences and mutual respect. The train lurched forward, and with it, my heart took flight. I was moving away from expectation, toward discovery. And somewhere in the blur of passing landscapes, I understood that luck isn't found, it's created by the brave choices we make when we dare to step off the beaten path.

The train's rhythmic clatter against the tracks became a soothing backdrop to my thoughts. There I was, body pressed into an unforgiving seat, my gaze fixed on the patchwork fields racing by. It seemed unreal—just days ago, I had been lounging in my backyard, laughter and the haze of youthful indiscretions filling the air. Now here I sat, a soldier swathed in the unfamiliarity of this new world, muscles still aching from training, my life's trajectory altered by the simple act of donning a uniform.

As towns slipped past, each with their own secrets and stories, a sense of wonder swelled within me. The realization that I was part of something larger than myself, larger than the small-town life I'd known, was both humbling and exhilarating. Life, it appeared, had its own plans for me, and it was leading me to places my backyard dreams could never touch.

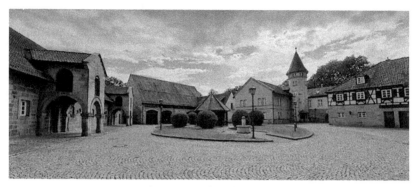

A picture taken in Rödental, Germany where
I spent much of my free time.

The guesthouse was modest but inviting, nestled in the heart of Roedental. The warmth within contrasted sharply with the crisp autumn air outside. Bernd spotted me almost immediately—a lone American amid the cadence of German conversation. His invitation to join him was accompanied by a smile that bridged any language barrier.

"American soldier?" he asked, his curiosity evident.

"Yes," I replied, feeling a kinship in his eagerness and the fact that he, too, was a soldier for the German army.

Bernd's friends shuffled to make room, their faces alight with genuine interest. They spoke in broken English, their words delivered with care, as if each sentence was a precious gift that they were presenting to me. We exchanged stories, laughter mingling with the clink of glasses, and I found myself enveloped in an unexpected camaraderie.

The colonel's words played like a mantra in my mind—they do love soldiers here, away from the shadow of the base. No hand reached out for payment when drinks were refilled or plates brought forth. Instead, they waved away my attempts, insisting it was their honor. Amid the backslapping and hearty cheers, I felt a gratitude

I struggled to articulate—for their generosity, for the colonel's wisdom, for this chance at a fresh start.

I made a silent vow then, surrounded by new friends in a country that once felt so alien. This village, this hidden gem amongst the rolling hills of Bavaria, would be my sanctuary. Here, amongst these few thousand souls, I would carve out a space where Bobby Quayle, the soldier, could become Bobby Quayle, the man.

My decision to spend my free time in this unassuming place was not just about escapism; it was about finding my own version of home. A home defined not by borders or language but by the open hearts of those who welcomed me.

As the weekend drew to a close, I carried with me more than memories—I carried the seeds of transformation. In that guesthouse, through gestures of goodwill and shared humanity, I discovered that fortune isn't merely stumbled upon. It's crafted through the choices we make—the brave, hopeful leaps into the unknown. And I, Bobby Quayle, was ready to jump.

CHAPTER 7

A Unique Opportunity

As I scrubbed the carbon off my M-16, the smell of gunmetal and CLP oil was as familiar as the determined resolve threading through my every action. My hands, steady and practiced, moved with a precision molded by repetition and necessity. I was a private first class now, each day a testament to the grit that had carried me from the uncertainty of youth to the structured life of a soldier.

"Private Quayle! Front and center!" The voice of authority sliced through the rhythmic sounds of maintenance. I looked up as the Battalion Command Sergeant Major strode purposefully toward us. His presence was like a sudden storm, commanding attention and respect without uttering another word.

I stood, placing my rifle on the table, and stepped forward. The military had honed my instincts for discipline; you responded to a call like that with urgency and expectation. Standing before him, I felt the weight of his gaze, an unspoken challenge to prove my worth in this sea of green and brown.

"Yes, Sergeant Major!" I acknowledged, meeting his eyes with the confidence I had cultivated not just in myself but also in the trust of those who had invested their time in me.

Bernd and his family came to mind—how they had welcomed me into their home, their culture. Our language lessons were more than mere exchanges of words; they were bridges between worlds. His English, colored with the soft Bavarian accent, improved with each visit, just as my German grew richer, infused with local idioms and expressions.

I found a strange joy in those sessions, the laughter when I stumbled over the harsher sounds, the pride when I finally captured the melody of their speech. They showed me a Germany untouched by the shadow of barracks and uniforms. In those moments, I was no longer Private Quayle. I was Bobby, the eager student, the honorary family member, someone more than the sum of his orders and duties.

"Private," the sergeant major's voice pulled me back to the present, "you've been making waves. That's good."

"Thank you, Sergeant Major," I replied, unsure where this was leading but ready to face it head-on. It wasn't just about following orders; it was about exceeding them, about showing that my motivations ran deeper than the surface, that my aspirations soared higher than the barracks' rooftops.

"Keep it up," he said, a brief nod acknowledging whatever he had seen in me. He turned then, leaving me amid my comrades with a sense of accomplishment that couldn't be polished away like the residue on my weapon.

As I returned to my task, I let the hope within me expand, fill the spaces of my being until there was no room for doubt. The future was an unfurling map, and I had only just begun to chart its course. With every lesson learned, every barrier crossed, I was crafting a narrative that defied expectations, one that spoke of resilience and the serendipity of luck.

The journey ahead would undoubtedly test me as all worthy journeys do. But the memories of warm smiles in a cozy guesthouse, the echoes of "*Danke*" and "*Bitte*" exchanged over dinner tables, they fortified me. I was building a life far from home, yet I had found home in unexpected places—in the hearts of people whose language I once could not speak, in the camaraderie of fellow soldiers, in the simple act of maintaining my rifle, knowing it was part of a larger story.

"Quayle," a fellow soldier called, snapping me back to the task at hand, "you gonna daydream your way through inspection?"

"Negative," I responded with a grin, picking up my rifle once more. This was my reality—a symphony of small tasks, each note contributing to a grander melody. And I was determined to play my part with all the zeal and fervor of a man who understood the value of each moment, each opportunity.

Yes, I would leave Germany one day, perhaps even lose my hard-earned accent, but I would carry with me the gifts of this land—the language, the friendships, and the unshakable belief that where you start is not where you have to end. Resilience isn't just about enduring; it's about thriving. And thrive I would, with hope as my compass and luck as my guide.

My heart pounded in rhythm with the sergeant major's steps as he paced before us, his boots thudding against the gravel like a metronome of authority. I rose to my feet, snapping into the position of parade rest with military precision, yet an unfamiliar tremor ran through my hands. A bead of sweat traced its way down my temple, born not from exertion but from the uncertainty swirling in my gut.

"Private Quayle! Front and center!" His voice rumbled across the field, part command, part challenge—a test of mettle that I could not afford to fail.

"Yes, Sergeant Major!" The words left my lips with a confidence I scarcely felt, hoping my voice would not betray the silent flutter of nerves beneath my starched uniform. As I stepped forward, the world seemed to narrow to the space between myself and the imposing figure before me.

"At ease, soldier," he instructed, his gaze appraising me with an intensity that suggested he was reading every line of my service record and every secret ambition held close to my chest.

"Private, I have heard some things about you, and I wanted to ask you a question." His tone softened just enough to carve a space for dialogue, yet it retained the edge of authority that commanded respect.

"Yes, Sergeant Major! What is the question?" My reply came quickly, the words lined up like soldiers on parade, ready to face whatever battle lay ahead.

The sergeant major leaned in, his eyes narrowing as if peering into the possibilities of my future. "You see," he explained, "I need a communications sergeant in Bravo Battery, and I asked three sergeants if they wanted the job. You know what they said?" He paused, allowing the weight of his words to settle over the assembled troops. "They said NO! Private, if you were a sergeant, what would you say?"

Time stretched and contracted around his question, a conundrum that demanded more than a simple yes or no. In that moment, I saw a crossroads laid out before me—one path paved with the safety of the known, the other a leap into the vast expanse of potential.

"Sergeant Major, my response would be, when do I start?" I responded, each word infused with the essence of hope, resilience, and an unwavering belief in seizing luck by the collar when it passes by. "I would welcome the challenge and serve with honor."

A flicker of approval crossed the sergeant major's craggy features, and in that affirmation, I felt the stirrings of something grand—an opportunity to prove my worth beyond the scope of rank and file. It was a chance to embody the ethos of those who taught me, from Bernd's patient guidance in language to the unnamed colonel whose wisdom whispered of embracing the new and unknown.

With a single phrase, "Good answer," he conveyed trust and expectation. "Now beat feet to the PX, get some Sergeant stripes, and report to Bravo Battery!" The weight of his words settled onto my shoulders, a heavy mantle that I could not let fall.

I glanced at the privates standing nearby, feeling their eyes on me as I made my next move. Handing my weapon to one of them, I turned and set off toward the PX, my heart beating in time with each step.

As I walked, the tremor in my hands gradually dissipated, replaced by a burning warmth of potential. This was no longer just about survival; it was about forging a path through uncharted territory. And I knew that where I stood now was only the beginning.

Arriving at the PX, I followed his instructions and purchased Sergeant stripes. As I affixed them to my uniform, I felt like shedding my old self and stepping into a new role. Each piece of my rifle that I dismantled represented another layer of myself being shed, while every reassembled component was a building block for the person I was becoming. Resilience wasn't just about enduring; it was about thriving.

With hope as my compass and luck as my guide, I set off to report to Bravo Battery. Every step forward was a testament to the commitment I had made—to myself and to those who believed in me. And as I marched on toward the unknown, I knew that nothing could stand in the way of my determination and resilience.

CHAPTER 8

EXCELLENCE AS A SOLDIER

Hoisting the last cardboard box over the threshold, I stepped into the domain that marked a new chapter—a single room in the barracks that was now solely mine. The space was sparse, the walls unadorned, and the air held a sterile chill common to military quarters, yet it resonated with a sense of independence. A luxury, really, for someone like me, only ten months deep into army life and already feeling the weight of responsibility more suited to seasoned shoulders. "Private First Class" was still fresh on my tongue, but here I was, not just a private anymore, though the echo of that title lingered. The small square window beckoned light into the room, casting a glow on the dull linoleum floor, inviting me to make this place something like a home. Shifting the box onto the floor, I considered where to unpack first, strategizing as if preparing for a silent battle against chaos.

The barracks were never going to win any hospitality awards; the communal showers and bathroom facilities were proof enough of that. They were scrubbed daily, yet no amount of bleach could disguise the wear of constant use by hundreds of soldiers. Disarray seemed to be an unwritten part of the code here—towels left abandoned on floors, sinks perpetually speckled with shaving cream and toothpaste. It wasn't filth, but it wasn't quite cleanliness either. To have a private room here was like finding an oasis in a desert of disorder. Sure, it was no five-star suite, but after sharing quarters with four unruly roommates in Charlie Battery, this was akin to an unexpected promotion in living standards. Here, at least, I could control the state of my surroundings. I could create a sliver of solitude amid the relentless hum of military life.

As I began to unpack, placing stacks of standard-issue clothing into the built-in locker, aligning each fold with precision, I allowed myself to bask in the quiet. There was something almost meditative about organizing my gear, a ritual that provided clarity and focus. It was in these moments of methodical tidying that I found peace, a rare commodity in the unpredictability of service. The room gradually took shape with each book, photo, and personal trinket finding its place.

My fingers brushed over the fabric of my uniform, tracing the insignia stitched into the material. Each thread was a testament to resilience, a marker of hope, a reminder of the serendipitous turns my life had taken since enlisting.

Outside my window, the world continued its cadence, boots marching in sync, voices calling out orders, the symphony of discipline and duty. Yet inside these four walls, I forged a pocket of tranquility, a space to breathe, to reflect, and to steel myself for whatever lay ahead. Here in this newly claimed sanctuary, I felt the stirrings of potential, the whisperings of a future paved with hard-won victories and lessons learned. There was a path unfolding before me, one that demanded grit and determination, and I was ready to walk it, step by deliberate step. After all, luck might have landed me this upgrade, but it would be resilience that carried me forward.

I leaned against the door frame, surveying the spartan simplicity of my new room. The stillness was a stark contrast to the bustling chaos I had left behind. The bare walls echoed with potential, eagerly awaiting the stories I would fill them with. Inhaling deeply, I could almost taste the fresh start that this space represented. It was mine and mine alone—an upgrade not just in living conditions but a symbol of the unexpected trajectory my military career had taken.

At eighteen, I was a sergeant in the making, though the title felt like a borrowed coat, oversized and unfamiliar. There were no grand ambitions in my mind when I enlisted; survival and service were the extent of my horizons. Yet here I was, standing on the cusp of leadership, bestowed with a responsibility that seemed to have sought me out rather than the other way around. The colonel's words at the airport came back to me as clear as if he were still standing there, imparting wisdom that now resonated with my own life: "If you are ever asked to perform any mission, no matter how difficult the task may seem at the time, you respond with 'Yes, sir' and perform that mission to the best of your ability."

His assurance was like a lighthouse beam cutting through the fog of self-doubt. How did he know? Perhaps some foresight is granted to those who have weathered many storms.

Unpacking the last of my boxes, I settled into the routine of organizing—something about setting order to physical objects gave me the illusion of control, a comforting lie in an unpredictable world. My hands methodically placed books on the shelf, each spine a chapter of who I was and what I might yet become. The promotion was unconventional, a bypassing of the usual rigmarole for something more fitting of the times. One day, I was Private First Class; the next I bore the makeshift mantle of an "Acting Jack Sergeant." My rank wasn't official, but the weight of it rested squarely on my shoulders. The command had seen fit to place their trust in me, to believe that I could rise to the occasion despite the greenness of my tenure. And perhaps they saw something else—a spark, a readiness to embrace the unforeseeable challenges that lay ahead.

It was a leap of faith, for them and for me. But isn't life itself a series of leaps, from one stone to another across the river of time? Some stones are slippery, others firm—and every so often, one finds a rock that feels destined to bear their weight. Staring at the uniform hanging neatly beside my bunk, the stripes seemed to shimmer with a challenge and a promise. They demanded excellence and whispered of futures yet to unfold. I reached out, fingers grazing the fabric, feeling the surge of hope that comes when luck and resilience intertwine. "Tomorrow," I murmured to myself, a quiet declaration in the solitude of my room. "Tomorrow, I step into these boots as a leader, ready to say, 'Yes sir,' ready to give my all."

I turned off the light, the darkness wrapping around me like a cocoon. In that moment, before sleep claimed me, I clung to the buoyant hope that tomorrow held. And in the deep recesses of my heart, where fear and courage danced their eternal waltz, I embraced the notion that maybe, just maybe, I was exactly where I was meant to be. As dawn broke over the barracks, I laced up my boots with meticulous care, each pull of the strings a reminder of the weight they now carried. The morning's chill seeped through the walls, whispering of tasks ahead and responsibilities newly borne. I stood before the mirror, adjusting the makeshift rank pinned upon my chest, an "Acting Jack Sergeant" staring back at me with eyes full of determination.

I met the day head-on, stepping out into the crisp air that seemed to sharpen my resolve. The communications section awaited me, four soldiers under my command, whose slumped shoulders and downcast eyes spoke volumes of their discontent. They were good men, no doubt, but disillusionment had taken root within them, growing like weeds in the cracks of their morale. They spoke in hushed tones about their disdain for this foreign land, their desire to return home, a sentiment I understood but could not afford to indulge.

The specter of the IG Inspection loomed large over us all. It was the kind of moment that would sift the chaff from the grain among the leadership, a crucible that could either forge or shatter a career. I felt the invisible weight of it settle on my shoulders, a mantle I had unwittingly volunteered to bear.

Bravo Battery's communications section needed more than just a leader; it needed a scapegoat, someone who could be the bulwark or the breach. The sergeant major's choice in selecting me, a greenhorn by any other name, was a stroke of tactical brilliance. If I succeeded, the accolades would be mine, along with the stripes that came with them. And if I failed, well, it was still a step up from where I began if I were demoted to Specialist E-4. A no-lose situation for the brass, perhaps, but for me, it was a gamble of the highest order.

As the day unfolded, I threw myself into the work, every cable checked, every report scoured for errors, every piece of equipment tested and retested. I could feel the scrutiny of my new charges. Their curiosity piqued as I navigated the labyrinth of our duties with unwavering focus. There was no room for doubt, no space for second-guessing. Each task completed was a brick laid in the foundation of our shared goal, each improvement a stitch in the fabric of a team slowly mending itself. The challenge that lay before us was monumental, but beneath the surface of my calm, a fire was stoked, fueled by the same resilience that had seen me through tougher times.

"Lead by example," the words echoed in my mind, a mantra that guided my actions, steady and sure. With each passing day, the transformation became tangible, not just in the readiness of our section, but in the subtle shift of attitudes among the men. Their conversations grew livelier, their laughter less hollow, a camaraderie rekindled from the embers of shared purpose.

In the quiet moments of reflection, when I allowed myself the luxury of introspection, I found hope nestled between the lines of duty and ambition. It was a fragile thing, easily crushed by the weight of expectation, yet it thrived, fed by the simple belief that luck favors the prepared. Tonight, as I lie in the darkness of my solitary room, the silence is a canvas for my thoughts. The journey ahead is fraught with uncertainty, but there is a beacon of possibility that refuses to dim. I close my eyes, embracing the promise of tomorrow and the resilience that has become my closest ally. "Step by step," I whisper to the night, "we will rise to meet the dawn." And in those words, I find the strength to believe that we will not only endure but prevail.

CHAPTER 9

LEADING BY EXAMPLE AND TRULY CARING

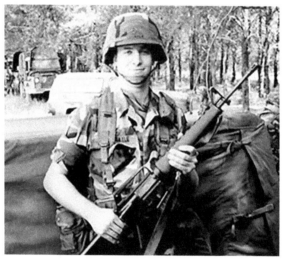

This was taken during field training in Grafenwohr, Germany
shortly after I was promoted to sergeant at the age of 18.

The chill of the German morning seeped through the walls of the
communications shop as I busied myself with a pile of paperwork
that seemed to multiply with every passing hour. My breath formed
tiny clouds in the frosty air, each one dissolving as quickly as my
doubts needed to. The clock was ticking, its hands sweeping away
the days I had left before the inspector general would scrutinize every
detail of my section. My fingers were stiff from the cold, dancing

over forms and checklists with mechanical precision. Yet beneath the numbness, a fire kindled in my belly—the unwavering resolve to see this mission through. I imagined the lines on those papers as the trenches I had to fortify, the numbers as soldiers standing at attention, ready for inspection.

I was so absorbed in the task that the sudden burst of laughter and clatter at the entrance startled me. The door swung open, letting in a gale that scattered documents into a whirlwind of chaos. Four figures stamped their boots free of snow, shaking off the winter's bite. They looked different somehow, their shoulders a touch less burdened, their eyes holding a flicker of something that resembled...hope?

"Morning, Sarge!" they chimed almost in unison, the warmth of their voices cutting through the cold. Before I could muster a response, they unloaded their unexpected bounty onto my desk. Two cases of quality German beer, beads of moisture glistening on the bottles like an offering of peace. For a moment, I stood there, the gravity of their gesture sinking in. It wasn't just about the beer; it was recognition, a silent acknowledgment of the solitary hours I'd poured into our shared goal.

A smile cracked my disciplined facade as I surveyed their expectant faces. "Let's save the brews for later," I said, the words feeling more like a promise than a command. "For now, here's what I need help with."

Their nods were eager, almost relieved as if they'd been waiting for the chance to dive into the trenches with me. Together, we set about reorganizing the chaos, their hands as steady as their newfound resolve. As we worked, the room grew warmer, not from the heat, which was still stubbornly absent, but from the sense of unity that stitched us together, patching the frayed edges of morale.

In those hours, surrounded by the hum of productivity and the occasional clink of tools, I glimpsed the future. There was a vision taking shape, one where failure was not a thread in the tapestry we wove. I saw us standing tall on the day of the inspection, not just as a section that passed but as a testament to what determination could accomplish against the odds. That Saturday marked a turning point, a pivot upon which the axis of our fate turned ever so slightly toward success. In the reflection of their earnest faces, I saw fragments of my own journey—the countless times I had been knocked down, only to rise again, stronger and more resolute.

As the day waned and shadows stretched across the room, I marveled at the progress we'd made, both in the tangible sense and within the hearts of those I led. We were building more than just a case for commendation; we were constructing a fortress of camaraderie, capable of withstanding any siege. "Step by step," I reminded myself as the last light of day surrendered to dusk. The road ahead was daunting, but luck has a way of siding with those who defy the odds. *With a crew like this*, I thought, *how could we be anything but lucky?*

The chill of the early morning air was brisk as it cut through the fibers of our dress green uniforms. We stood in formation outside the communications shop, a line of soldiers bound by a singular mission. Every crease in our attire was sharp, every polished boot reflecting the pale light of dawn. The hum of anticipation buzzed through us, electric and infectious. I scanned the faces of my team, each one a mirror of the dedication that had brought us to this pivotal moment. My soldiers' expressions were etched with the same blend of nerves and confidence that I felt swirling in my gut. Months of relentless preparation, of turning wrenches and poring over schematics, of drilling protocols until they were etched in our minds—all of it led to this. "Today, we prove ourselves," I whispered under my breath, more a vow than an affirmation.

As the brass approached, their medals glinting in the burgeoning daylight, my heart pounded a fierce rhythm. This was it—the inspection that would either forge or shatter our futures. Yet standing there amid my comrades, I knew we had done everything within our power to tip the scales in our favor. Our boots crunched in unison as we snapped to attention, the sharp sound slicing through the silence. The inspectors moved through our ranks, their scrutiny meticulous, as they examined every detail of our work. Time stretched, taut and endless, as we awaited their verdict. And then success—sweet and resounding. Not only did we pass the inspection, but we had outshone the Battalion Communications section itself. It was a victory hard-earned and savored by each one of us who had poured soul and sweat into the endeavor.

The following Monday, the atmosphere in the shop was charged with a different kind of electricity. It was the buzzing of pride, the kind that resonates deep in your chest and lights up your every fiber. My commander, the first sergeant, and command sergeant major entered with commendations in hand, their faces alight with respect that mirrored our own sense of accomplishment. "Attention to orders," came the call, and we stiffened, our chests swelling with pride.

One by one, my soldiers stepped forward to receive their achievement medals, tokens of their skill and perseverance. When my turn came, the weight of the commendation medal in my hands felt like holding a piece of the sun—warm, radiant, and powerful. "Congratulations, Sergeant," the command sergeant major said, his voice carrying the gravity of our shared journey. "Your leadership made this possible."

I looked down at the stripes on my arm, their significance now heightened beyond measure. Wearing them, I no longer felt the shadow of doubt that once clung to me like a second skin. I was a sergeant, not by default or desperation but by merit and the unwavering faith of those who followed me.

In the quiet that followed the ceremony, I stood before the window, gazing out at the barracks that had become both home and battleground. A warm glow settled in my chest, a beacon of hope that whispered of future challenges and triumphs yet to come. "Step by step," I murmured, the reflection of my stripes in the glass a testament to resilience and luck and to the belief that even the most daunting odds can be defied. The echo of their departure had barely faded when the Sergeant Major leaned in, his presence both imposing and reassuring.

"Are you ready for the promotion board so we can make those official?" he whispered, nodding toward the stripes adorning my sleeve. "Roger, Sergeant Major," I replied, the words firm and resolute—a reflection of newfound confidence rather than bravado. The stripes felt like a covenant between me and the future I was determined to forge.

As the leadership's footsteps receded into silence, I turned to face my soldiers, their faces etched with the fatigue of duty well-executed but also with something less definable. A quiet unease, perhaps, or the restless stirrings of discontent. "All right, everyone," I began, gripping the edge of a metal desk that had seen too many years and too many wars. "There's one thing left to do that might be more important than the inspection we just passed." Curiosity flickered in their eyes, a shared moment of wondering what could possibly eclipse our recent victory. "I understand the four of you hate Germany and can't wait to leave—is that true?"

The question hung in the air, an invitation for honesty.

Their affirmations came readily, laced with grievances about the monotony of base life and the suffocating sameness of the surrounding city. It was as if they were echoing the colonel's words, giving voice to a collective yearning for something beyond the confines of duty and discipline. I listened, each reason resonating with the same sense of confinement I'd once felt. But where there was confinement, there was also the potential for release. In their words, I heard not just complaints but a challenge—a mission of a different sort that beckoned me with the same urgency as any orders from above.

It was then, in the midst of this reckoning, that hope took seed. Here was an opportunity not only to lead but to inspire, to show them that the world outside these walls was as much a part of their service as the uniforms we wore. "Listen up," I said, my voice carrying the weight of conviction. "We've got work to do, and it's not just about inspections and medals. It's about living—really living—in this place that fate has dropped us. Let's find out what Germany has to offer beyond the barbed wire and the barracks."

A murmur of assent rippled through them, tentative but growing stronger. And with that, I knew that the next chapter of our story was just beginning—one where resilience would be our compass and hope our guide as we navigated the unfamiliar terrain of foreign streets and open skies. In that moment, luck seemed to be on our side as it had been since I first set foot in this country, and I was resolved to chase it as far as it would take us.

I led them on the same journey I had once taken by train, through the rolling green hills and quaint villages of the German countryside. As we sat in the train car, sipping on cold, refreshing German beer and chatting about the successful inspection we had just completed, we were surrounded by picturesque views of idyllic landscapes. The melodious tunes of Billy Joel's music filled the air from our trusty boom box as we chugged toward our final destination: Coburg, Germany.

This bustling city was larger than the quiet village of Roedental where my secret sanctuary lay hidden. I wanted to spare its residents from any disturbance, so I chose to bring my soldiers here instead. It was a chance for them to see why Germany was not such a bad place after all, with its charming mix of old-world charm and modern city life.

The crisp morning air held a tinge of anticipation as I strode toward the promotion board room, my boots clicking in rhythm on the polished floor. The corridor seemed to stretch longer with each step, mirroring the journey that had brought me to this pivotal point. My mind was a whirlwind of regulations, procedures, and potential questions, each one meticulously reviewed during the endless hours of preparation that had consumed my nights. As the door swung open, I stepped into the room where my fate would be decided. A panel of four first sergeants and the command sergeant major, their faces etched with years of service, scrutinized me as I presented myself. There was no room for doubt, only the confidence that I had forged in the crucible of leadership and responsibility. With every response, I felt the stripes on my arm grow heavier, imbued with the promise of what was to come.

"Congratulations, Sergeant," the board president finally said, his voice resonating with approval. In that moment, the trials and triumphs of the past months coalesced into a single, staggering reality—I had succeeded. As I exited the room, the weight lifted, replaced by an electric surge of pride and purpose. Time passed in a blur, the days marked by training and the quiet satisfaction of knowing my efforts were recognized. And then, under the gaze of the entire battalion, I stood tall as the rank of sergeant was officially bestowed upon me.

At eighteen years old, adorned with medals that glittered in the sunlight, I was a testament to what could be achieved through sheer determination and relentless drive. The commendations and achievements were not just decorations; they were symbols of the resilience and fortitude that had defined my service.

But it was the unexpected summons from the battalion commander that brought a new dimension to my journey. With a salute that was both an acknowledgment and a commitment, I listened intently as the lieutenant colonel outlined the mission that awaited me. His words didn't just convey an assignment; they entrusted me with a responsibility that extended far beyond my own aspirations. In the silent affirmation of my readiness, I understood that this was more than a mere task—it was a chance to prove that the seeds of hope planted in adversity could blossom into something extraordinary. This was my opportunity to demonstrate that luck was not a fleeting chance but a reward for those who dared to embrace the challenges laid before them.

The chill of the room bit at my skin as I stood rigid, my boots planted like roots into the polished floor of the battalion commander's office. The air was thick with a sense of occasion; the kind that heralds change and whispers of new horizons. My heart drummed a cadence in my chest, syncopated with the silent mantra that had become my creed: perform the mission to the best of your ability.

"Yes, sir," I said, my voice a steadfast echo of the commitment I carried within. There was no room for doubt or hesitation. It was the response of a soldier ready to cross the next threshold, whatever it might be. The colonel's gaze held a weight of expectation as he unfolded before me the contours of my new assignment.

"We need a sergeant in Intelligence," he began, his words painting a picture of the uncharted path ahead. My mind raced, piecing together fragments of training and experience, each a stepping stone I had traversed to reach this point. His assessment of my record, the commendation wrought from the crucible of leadership and the quiet triumphs behind closed doors—it all led here, to this moment.

"Your performance thus far has been exemplary," he continued. And with those words, I felt the swell of hope rise within me, not born of naivety but forged in the fires of relentless dedication. I was more than just a name on a file; I was the sum of countless hours and unwavering resolve. The lieutenant colonel's revelation of the counterintelligence operation unfurled a new canvas, a challenge steeped in shadows and intrigue. Yet within its folds lay an opportunity—a testament to the belief that had been placed in me by those who commanded my fate. As the gravity of the mission settled upon me, I recalled Sergeant Lisa Martinez's unspoken lessons: the strength she wielded with ease, her quick wit cutting through uncertainty, her loyalty an anchor in the storm. She was the embodiment of resilience, and now, so must I be.

In the stillness of the commander's office, I found myself peering into the future, a mosaic of potential and promise. This was not the end of a journey but the beginning of an ascent, with every step a chance to embody the ideals I had been taught. Stepping outside, the morning sunlight spilled over the barracks, casting long shadows that stretched out like the years that lay before me. In that light, the world seemed vast and filled with endless possibility. And there, with a steady breath and a heart brimming with anticipation, I walked forward—an instrument of hope in a theater of the unseen.

Luck had never been a random gift; it was the offspring of courage and conviction. As I moved toward my new role in Intelligence, I understood that luck was waiting to be claimed by those who dared to grasp it. And so with a spirit buoyed by purpose, I would meet this next chapter head-on, ready to carve a legacy from the unknown with resilience as my guide and hope as my compass.

The crisp morning air bit at my cheeks as I strode across the base, the weight of the battalion commander's words settling in my bones. The world around me hummed with the routine of military life, but today, it felt like a backdrop to the mission that lay ahead—a mission steeped in shadows and woven with espionage. "Roger, sir." My voice was steady, a contrast to the adrenaline coursing through my veins. East German agents were out there, their methods insidious and varied, preying on the vulnerabilities of soldiers. Bribery, extortion, seduction—the tools of a war fought without guns or tanks but with whispered secrets and traded loyalties.

My training had covered this, yet knowledge was one thing; facing the reality was another. I remembered the colonel's advice, his words a guiding star in the murky world I was about to navigate. "Avoid the local girls near the base," he'd said. "Their allure could be a trap, a sweetly sung siren's call leading to ruin." I had taken those warnings to heart, understanding the stakes of such fraternization.

The commander's gaze pierced through me, discerning, as he revealed the crux of my assignment. "Well, Sergeant, you're the ideal candidate." His voice held an edge of confidence, a belief in me that I was still learning to accept. Out of uniform, I might appear as a green young soldier, still wet behind the ears—easy prey for those hunting secrets. But appearances can deceive. I knew the local tongue; German flowed from my lips as easily as English, a secret weapon in a silent battle. "We know that you're not so wet behind the ears," he said, a hint of a smile betraying his composed facade, "but that's our secret."

I left the commander's office feeling as though I had stepped onto an invisible battlefield, where every conversation could be laced with danger and each new acquaintance might harbor ulterior motives. Yet amid these thoughts, there was no room for doubt. Uncertainty was a luxury I could ill afford. The path before me required resilience, the same quality I'd seen in Sergeant Lisa Martinez, her quick wit cutting through uncertainty, her loyalty an anchor in the storm. She was the embodiment of resilience, and now, so must I be.

In the stillness of the commander's office, I found myself peering into the future, a mosaic of potential and promise. This was not the end of a journey but the beginning of an ascent, with every step a chance to embody the ideals I had been taught. Stepping outside, the morning sunlight spilled over the barracks, casting long shadows that stretched out like the years that lay before me. In that light, the world seemed vast and filled with endless possibility. And there, with a steady breath and a heart brimming with anticipation, I walked forward—an instrument of hope in a theater of the unseen. Luck had never been a random gift; it was the offspring of courage and conviction. As I moved toward my new role in Intelligence, I understood that luck was waiting to be claimed by those who dared to grasp it.

And so with a spirit buoyed by purpose, I would meet this next chapter head-on, ready to carve a legacy from the unknown with resilience as my guide and hope as my compass. The wind carried a chill that belied the crispness of the day as I stepped outside, my boots crunching on the gravel with an assertive cadence. The mission ahead loomed large—a game of cat and mouse with stakes far beyond what the eye could see. I was to be bait, a role that felt at odds with the uniform I wore, yet it was a mantle I accepted with the gravity it deserved.

In the past, I might have balked at the idea of being seen as young and naive, but now I understand the power in underestimation. As I walked through the streets, each step was measured and purposeful, for I carried within me the knowledge that every encounter could be the veil before a clandestine dance. With my German language skills tucked away like a hidden blade, I was more than the facade they would perceive. I watched the people around me, their faces etched with the ordinary concerns of life. My gaze lingered on nothing in particular, but my mind was alight with strategies and scenarios. It was a mental chess game, one where I had been given the opportunity to checkmate those who sought to exploit our vulnerabilities.

Training as an intelligence analyst added layers to my perception, sharpening my instincts. Codes and signals became second nature, and I learned to read the subtle tells of those who might not be what they seem. Each briefing, each drill honed my senses until I could almost feel the pulse of information coursing unseen through the air, a symphony of secrets waiting to be deciphered. The thrill of the challenge invigorated me, lending a buoyancy to my stride. Hope coursed through my veins, a hope not just for personal success but for the safeguarding of my fellow soldiers, my friends, the very ideals we stood to protect. There was a certain poetry in the notion that by pretending to be vulnerable, I was, in fact, guarding against vulnerability itself.

Luck, I mused, had become a silent partner in my endeavors. Yet it was not the fickle hand of fate but rather the product of preparation meeting the precipice of opportunity. I had been given a chance to make a difference, to prove that resilience could be both shield and sword. As I walked the cobblestone paths threading through the quaint German town, I allowed myself to soak in the beauty of the old-world architecture, the laughter of children playing in the distance. It was a stark contrast to the shadowy role I now played—a reminder that beneath the surface of tranquility, danger often lurked.

But there was a steadfast sense of hope in me, a burgeoning belief that the work I was doing mattered, that it contributed to something greater than myself. And so with each breath, each step, each day that passed, I embraced the mission, the risk, and the chance to serve with unwavering commitment. It was here, in this intricate dance of espionage, that I found a new facet of myself—a resilience born of duty and a hope that gleamed like a beacon through the fog of war. This was my crucible, and I would emerge tempered and steadfast, ready to face whatever lay ahead with a heart fortified by the trials overcome and the successes yet to come.

The clink of beer glasses chimed like a cacophony of bells, each toast a reverberation through the crowded room and into my chest. In the heart of Roedental, the local hangout brimmed with life—a farewell to rival any storied Oktoberfest celebration. The scent of lager and hearty German fare mingled in the air as laughter and the thump of boots dancing on tables set the rhythm for the night. I watched, a smile tugging at my lips, as my friends—those steadfast allies in a foreign land—belted out American tunes with heavy accents. They stumbled over words but not spirit, their voices rising in a boisterous homage that transcended language barriers.

In this jubilant chaos, I found a bittersweet solace. These were the people who had seen me grow from an unsure youth to a confident sergeant, the ones who'd stood by me through trials that tested my mettle, through days when the weight of leadership rested uneasily on my shoulders. Yet even as we reveled, there was an undercurrent of finality that no amount of drink could wash away. Each clasp on the shoulder, every shared joke, was tinged with the silent acknowledgment of our parting. I was leaving behind more than just a place; I was saying goodbye to a part of myself that had been forged in the camaraderie and challenges of this foreign landscape.

As the night waned, the revelry did not. We danced until our feet ached, sang until our voices cracked. And when the hour grew late, and the festivities wound down, my heart swelled with gratitude for these friendships that would linger long after my military service ended.

I stepped outside, the cool air sobering my senses. Turning back, I etched the scene into memory—the outline of the tavern windows glowing against the dark sky, the silhouettes of my friends as they continued to celebrate inside. With a deep breath, I felt a quiet resolve settle within me. This chapter was closing, but it wasn't the end of my story. It was simply the turning of a page, an impetus to carry forward the lessons and love from this time and place. My departure from Germany was not just a transfer of duty stations; it was a commencement of sorts, the start of a new journey fueled by the resilience and hope fostered here. As I walked away from the laughter still spilling from the tavern, I carried with me the warmth of a sendoff only Germans could provide—a fitting tribute to the years that had shaped the man I had become. As I packed the last of my belongings into the olive drab duffel bag, I felt the weight of the impending departure settle on my shoulders. The room that had been my sanctuary—the walls adorned with photos of Therese and me, the small tokens of affection we'd exchanged—now stood starkly empty, the remnants of our shared memories tucked away in boxes.

Therese's smile haunted me as I latched the bag closed. We had met by chance during a weekend outing to Roedental, her laughter like a melody that cut through the chatter of the busy street fair. Our connection was instant, a bond that deepened over countless evenings spent strolling along the winding streets, sharing dreams beneath the benevolent gaze of the stars. But as my orders drew near, a chasm grew between us—a rift born not of anger or betrayal but of an unspoken understanding that our paths were diverging. She clung to the cobbled lanes and timber-framed houses of her homeland, while my life marched to the cadence of duty's call. In the end, the love that had blossomed between us wilted under the harsh reality that I must go where the army sends me.

With one final glance around the barracks room, I slung the bag over my shoulder and stepped out into the brisk morning air. Germany had been more than just a posting; it was the anvil upon which my character had been forged. From a green private to a decorated sergeant, I had grown into my skin here, discovering the steel in my spine and the compassion in my heart.

The rumble of the C-130's engines filled the tarmac as I climbed aboard, finding a seat among the ranks of soldiers, each lost in their own thoughts. My hand reached for the comfort of music, the familiar shape of my Walkman a welcome distraction from the swirl of emotions. As Billy Joel's "Vienna" began to play, the gentle piano mingling with his poignant words, I gazed through the porthole at the retreating landscape.

Tears, unbidden yet unabashed, traced paths down my cheeks as the German countryside receded below. It was not just a farewell to a place but to a chapter of life that had shaped me indelibly. Through service and sacrifice, love and loss, I had found the resilience to endure and the hope to aspire.

As the aircraft ascended, climbing higher until the towns became mere specks, I felt a sense of purpose swell within me. Each trial faced, each obstacle overcome, had led me to this moment—a culmination of experiences that would serve as the foundation for all the adventures yet to come. With the horizon stretched out before me, I was ready for whatever lay ahead, carrying with me the lessons of the past and the promise of tomorrow.

CHAPTER 10

BECOMING A CIVILIAN AGAIN

The Georgia sun beat down like a hammer, its heat relentless as I stepped off the bus onto the scalding pavement of Fort Benning. It was a stark contrast to the cooler, temperate climes of Germany, where my military life had been, up until that moment, defined. The air was thick with humidity, wrapping around me like a heavy blanket, a tactile reminder that this was my final station before I reentered civilian life.

Sweat already beading on my brow, I squinted against the bright light and surveyed the sprawling base. It teemed with energy, the pulse of boots hitting the ground in unison, young soldiers being forged into warriors under the watchful eyes of their drill sergeants. Fort Benning: the birthplace of infantrymen, a proving ground for the elite Airborne Army Rangers and Green Berets. But for me, it was the backdrop to a countdown, the last pages of a chapter I was ready to close.

At twenty-one, the rest of my life loomed large before me, a canvas blank and beckoning. There was something thrilling about the uncertainty, the boundless potential of the "real world" beyond the regimented confines of military order. My decision not to reenlist had settled in my chest with a weight that felt surprisingly like freedom, not the heft of trepidation I'd expected.

I trudged toward the barracks, my duffel bag slung over one shoulder, a physical manifestation of the journey I'd undergone. From enlistee to seasoned soldier, each stitch and patch on that worn canvas told a story of resilience, a testament to the trials overcome.

The dust of foreign lands still clung to it, grains of history that whispered of the past.

As I walked, my thoughts drifted. What would life hold for me once I shed the identity of Sergeant Bobby Quayle? Could I adapt, find purpose without the structure the army provided? The thought gripped me but not with fear—more like the anticipation one feels before diving into the unknown depths of an ocean. I knew challenges awaited, but the possibilities sparked a fire within, a flame fueled by hope and the hunger for a new beginning.

There were no grand farewells or bugle calls to mark my impending departure. This transition was a personal affair, quiet and introspective. Still, I couldn't help but feel like Lady Luck had her eye on me, perhaps favoring the boldness of my choice to embark on a different path, away from the security of a guaranteed career in the military.

The base sounds faded into a muted cacophony as I turned inward, considering the traits that had carried me through my service: determination, adaptability, the willingness to face adversity head-on. These, I realized, were the very tools I'd need to forge success in civilian life. And they were tools I possessed in abundance.

Fort Benning was not an end but a gateway, and as I continued to walk, my heart lifted. I felt the shackles of routine begin to loosen, the future calling out to me with a siren's song. Whether it led to triumph or trial, it was mine to seize. With every step, I left behind the shadow of who I'd been, stepping closer to the man I was meant to become—a man ready to take on the world, come what may.

The weight of the Georgia heat pressed down upon me as I marched toward the Battalion Commander's office, the air thick with the scent of sun-scorched earth and anticipation. This was no ordinary day at Fort Benning; the relentless sun seemed to underscore the gravity of what was about to unfold. My steps were measured, each one a deliberate march toward a future unknown.

"Enter," came the authoritative voice from within as I knocked on the solid door. The room was stark, functional, filled with the hum of an overworked air conditioner trying to combat the sweltering heat. As I stood before the Battalion Commander, his gaze bore into me, as if trying to gauge my readiness for the words he was about to impart.

"Sergeant," he began, his voice steady as granite, "you're going to be one of the Battalion COMSEC Custodians."

The role hit me like a jolt of electricity—unexpected, powerful, transforming.

"You will shoulder the responsibility for our communications security. This includes our encryption codes and, critically, the nuclear launch codes."

I could feel the pulse in my neck, thumping with the realization of the trust being placed in my hands. It was an assignment that I had never fathomed, yet here it was, laid out before me as a testament to my service and the top-secret clearance level I'd earned through diligence and discipline. A silent acknowledgment that I was more than just another soldier; I was a guardian of national secrets.

"Understood, sir," I replied, my voice betraying none of the inner turmoil that this revelation had sparked. In partnership with Captain Grandston, I would become a sentinel for the most potent and terrifying weapons known to mankind. The magnitude of such a task wasn't lost on me. It was a burden I was determined to bear with honor.

As I left the commander's office, my mind raced with the practicalities of my new role. Yet beneath the surface-level concerns about protocols and procedures, there lay a deeper current—a sense of purpose reignited. The military had honed my skills, but it was my resilience and hope that made me thrive in adversity.

With every step away from the office, I felt the convergence of my past experiences and future potential. The boy who once looked up at the sky dreaming of what lay beyond now held in trust the very mechanisms that could rain fire from above. It was a sobering thought, one that anchored me firmly in the present while propelling me forward.

This was more than just a final duty; it was a pinnacle of responsibility, a capstone to my time in uniform. And though my path was set to diverge into civilian life, I realized how intertwined my journey had been with the fabric of fate. Chance encounters, serendipitous assignments—they all led me here, to this moment, standing at the crossroads of history and destiny.

A newfound clarity settled within me as I prepared to meet Captain Grandston. There was pride, yes, but also a profound reverence for the gravity of our shared duty. We would stand as vigilant custodians, keepers of peace through the paradox of power. And when the time came to lay down that mantle, I would step into the world beyond the gates of Fort Benning transformed, ready to embrace the myriad opportunities that awaited with unwavering hope and the luck that had always seemed to follow those willing to carve their own path.

I stepped onto the parched Georgia soil, a world away from the cool mists of Germany, and I couldn't help but marvel at fate's hand. As if by some cosmic jest, Mr. Magoo strikes again, echoing in my inner monologue with an incredulous chuckle. Who would have thought that a young man, eager to explore life beyond the olive drab confines of the military, would find himself entrusted with such a monumental task?

The news of my assignment had hit me like a bolt from the blue—COMSEC Custodian, guardian of codes that held the weight of worlds. The responsibility was a staggering one; it felt as though I were being handed the keys to Pandora's box, tasked with ensuring its contents remained a secret sealed away from prying eyes.

My office, if you could call it that, was more of a fortress within a fortress. The Battalion Commander wasn't exaggerating when he detailed the security measures. Each step toward the door of this clandestine chamber resonated against the hum of activity outside. My boots clicked on the concrete as I approached what would be my domain for the remainder of my service.

Captain Grandston, already there, gave a curt nod. We both knew the drill without exchanging a word. Our hands moved independently yet synchronized, each turning a dial until the last click signified an alignment of trust and duty. It took our combined strength to pull open the vault-like door, revealing a space that promised no secrets could ever escape its confines.

Inside, the walls encased us in lead and steel—a silent testament to the lengths taken to protect the nation's most sensitive information. The air was heavy, not just with the mustiness of a room designed to keep out more than just the elements but with the palpable sense of importance that clung to every surface, every encrypted machine, every codebook stored within.

As the door sealed behind us, the silence enveloped me. Here, in this bunker beneath the earth, I realized the capstone of my military career was not just a culmination of service but a bridge to my future self. This role was a trust, a final test of my resilience, demanding a vigilance I knew was woven into the very fabric of my being.

I allowed myself a moment to absorb the gravity. The boy who once dreamed of untold possibilities was now the man responsible for safeguarding them. It was in this reflective solitude, surrounded by the tools of cryptic warfare, that a hopeful resolve blossomed within me. No matter where life's journey would lead next, the fortitude and luck which had carried me through to this point would surely not abandon me now.

With hope as my steadfast companion, I stood ready to embrace whatever lay ahead, carrying the lessons of the past and the promise of tomorrow. Yes, these walls spoke of secrecy and power, but to me, they whispered of change—the end of one chapter and the beginning of another. And so with a deep breath and a firm resolve, I accepted my charge in this quiet bastion, knowing full well that the true strength of any code lies not in its complexity but in the integrity of those who hold it.

The finality of the heavy vault door clanging shut behind me echoed a definitive end to my active-duty service. I stepped out from the bunker's shadow into the glaring Georgia sun, feeling it on my face like a herald of the new life awaiting me beyond the confines of Fort Benning. It was in this sun-soaked silence that I felt the weightlessness of freedom for the first time; the rigid structure of military life slowly dissipating like the morning mist.

Over those last two years, the challenge of safeguarding top-secret codes had been both a privilege and a crucible, honing my sense of responsibility and further tempering my resolve. Each day was met with strict routines and meticulous checks, the importance of our task never allowing complacency. There was pride in that, a quiet honor in knowing the security of many rested in the integrity of my hands. Yet as each day drew to a close, the distant call of civilian life grew louder, more insistent, a siren song of opportunity that promised a different kind of fulfillment.

The practical side of me, the one sculpted by years of training and experience, knew the transition wouldn't be seamless. It was this foresight that led me to enlist in the Ohio National Guard. A safety net woven from threads of caution and prudence, ensuring that if the winds of chance failed to carry me where I hoped, the fall wouldn't break me.

Then came liberation day. Discharge papers in hand, I walked away from my post not with trepidation but with an eagerness that bordered on impatience. The youthful naïveté that once fueled dreams of grandeur had matured into a measured anticipation for what lay ahead. I was no longer the boy who had enlisted with wide-eyed wonder; six years had chiseled away at that version of myself, leaving in its wake a man shaped by discipline, enriched by friendships, and tested by trials both expected and unforeseen.

The sun hadn't even kissed the horizon good morning when I sprang out of bed, a live wire of anticipation. My pulse thrummed in my ears, a symphony to accompany the birth of my first day as a civilian. The stiff military sheets felt alien now, relics of a life I was leaving behind. Six long years had passed—years of discipline, camaraderie, and growth that had transformed me from a boy with more questions than answers into a man with purpose.

I dressed quickly, favoring comfort over formality for my journey home. *Home*—the word tasted sweet and foreign on my tongue. It was time to rediscover what it meant, to build it anew with the pieces of myself I'd salvaged and sculpted during my service.

Standing in the empty barracks room, I felt the weight of memories press against the walls—laughter, orders barked in the dead of night, boots thudding in unison. But today, they were just echoes growing fainter by the second, drowned out by the call of freedom.

With a deep breath, I shouldered my duffel bag, its contents a mosaic of my military life. Dog tags jangled a soft farewell as I crossed the threshold for the last time, closing the door on an era.

Outside, my blue 1979 Chevy Camaro Z-28 waited, a chariot ready to whisk me back to a world I'd left behind. She was a beauty, all sleek lines and promises of the open road. Every item I owned was carefully stowed in her belly. Yesterday's farewells still lingered in the air, bittersweet, but necessary. There was no space for looking back, not when life was impatiently tapping its foot, waiting for me to catch up.

Sliding behind the wheel, my hands found their familiar grooves on the steering wheel, and I felt a kinship with this machine. We were both built for more than what we'd been given, hungry for the miles yet to be traveled. I turned the key, and she roared to life, a fierce declaration of our departure. The engine's rumble vibrated through me, mirroring my own restless energy.

As I eased the Camaro onto the road, I offered a silent salute to Fort Benning. This place, with its sweltering heat and relentless training, had sharpened me like steel on a whetstone. It had tested me, breaking me down only to rebuild me stronger. And now, armed with resilience and hope, I was ready to carve out my place in the vast unknown.

The drive ahead was long, but the distance felt trivial compared to the internal journey I'd already traveled. Ohio lay ahead, its familiar landscapes etched in my mind like a postcard from another life. Yet I knew I wouldn't be returning to the same place I'd left. How could I, when I was no longer the same person?

But before I left, there was one more thing left to do. Say goodbye to my fellow soldiers in a "proper" way.

The morning sun was already beating down, casting long shadows across the parade ground as I slipped behind the wheel of my Camaro. The engine idled, a low growl promising escape and adventure. I glanced over at the soldiers in formation—a tableau of discipline and camaraderie that had been my world for so long. Their faces were stoic, but their eyes betrayed them, some sparkled with mischief, others with unspoken yearnings.

With a deep breath, I gripped the steering wheel, feeling its familiar leather against my palms. This wasn't just any departure; it was my declaration of independence. My foot pressed down on the accelerator, the car responding with eager ferocity. The tires bit into the asphalt, and we lurched forward, tires squealing and plumes of dark smoke marking the beginning of my journey.

As the formation of soldiers came into view, I couldn't help but crack a grin. It stretched wide, unbidden, fueled by the thrill of what lay ahead. In a moment of reckless abandon, I raised my hand through the open window, my middle finger proudly extended. It was a salute of sorts—an irreverent farewell to the past.

"Good luck, you fucker!" The shout cut through the din of my revving engine, and laughter rippled through the ranks. They saluted back, some with their own gestures, others with smiles that mirrored mine. For a moment, our shared defiance bound us tighter than any military oath ever could.

I couldn't help but pause at the threshold of the base, taking a moment to look back. This wasn't just a farewell to a place or a profession; it was an acknowledgment of transformation. The barracks, the parade grounds, and even the mess hall—each held memories that were now chapters of a story I was ready to continue elsewhere.

Freedom's grasp was warm as I left the base and headed out into the embrace of a future unscripted. Home in Ohio beckoned with the allure of the unknown, a blank canvas on which I could paint the American dream as I saw it. Perhaps a quaint house with a white picket fence, a loving family, and a career that would make use of the skills and values instilled in me by the army.

As I drove away, the rearview mirror reflected the shrinking image of my former life, a life lived with dedication and distinction. Ahead, the road unwound toward the horizon—a symbol of the journey that awaited, filled with hope and ripe with possibilities. My heart beat with the rhythm of opportunity, each mile traveled a step closer to a new beginning. Yes, there would be challenges; yes, there might be setbacks. But I carried within me the resilience of a soldier, the adaptability of a survivor, and the optimism of a dreamer.

"Let's see what you've got in store for me," I whispered to the world beyond, a world I was now ready to claim as my own.

As the base shrank behind me, disappearing in the rearview mirror, my thoughts turned inward. The rigidity of basic training had once chafed, but now I saw it as the anvil upon which I was shaped. Germany, with its ancient streets and vibrant culture, had expanded my horizons, while Europe's winding paths had taught me the joy of exploration.

I thought of my drill sergeant, Lisa Martinez, her quick wit always cutting through tension like a knife; of Bernd, whose laughter was a balm to the soul in the darkest of times. Bonds forged in adversity are the strongest, they say. If that's true, then I carry with me an unbreakable chain of fellowship that will endure whatever comes next.

Miles unfolded before me, the road a gray ribbon stretching into the distance. The hum of the engine was a steady companion as I navigated the highways that would lead me home. Ohio felt both near and infinitely distant—a place of memories, not quite ready to welcome the man I had become.

I didn't have a grand plan, no meticulously charted course. But isn't that the beauty of it? Life's rich tapestry is woven not from certainty but from the willingness to face the uncertain. I had my skills, my drive, and a resilience honed by years of service. That would have to be enough.

"Let's find our path," I murmured to the Camaro as if she were a trusted confidant. She responded with a surge of power, as eager as I to discover what lay beyond the horizon. Together, we raced toward a future painted with hope and the promise of new beginnings. The unknown beckoned, and with every mile, I embraced it more fully.

There would be challenges, no doubt. Yet as the familiar landscape began to change, signaling my return to civilian life, I felt a sense of anticipation. Home awaited, not as a destination but as a starting point. And I, a soldier no longer, was ready to answer its call.

The Ohio sun filtered through the blinds, throwing lines of light across the bare walls of my new apartment. It was a stark contrast to the cramped and orderly quarters I'd grown used to in the barracks.

Here, space stretched before me, filled only with potential. The air felt different, thick with the scent of fresh paint and possibilities.

I had wasted no time getting my feet under me. In just two short weeks, life had propelled me from the structured regimen of the military to the sprawling unpredictability of civilian existence. I found myself employed, housed, and surprisingly involved.

It started with the job—a position that seemed trivial compared to the high-stakes responsibilities I'd shouldered in uniform. Nevertheless, it was a foothold, and for now, that's all I needed. "What makes you think that you can be a security guard?" the security chief had asked, skepticism laced within his tone. His ignorance of my past was almost comical.

"Sir," I said, leaning back in the metal folding chair, "I've guarded more than just fences and walls. I've held the safety of nations between vigilant eyes and steady hands." His eyebrows had lifted slightly, the hint of a challenge in my voice not lost on him. "If I can keep nuclear launch codes safe from those who wish us harm, then I surely can manage the security of your mall."

"Okay, then, I guess you're hired," he responded after a pause. And just like that, my weekdays were booked, patrolling under fluorescent skies, watching over a citadel of commerce rather than one of deadly force.

Next came the apartment—a modest one-bedroom that I could afford on my own. No roommates, no shared bunks, just me and whatever future I chose to build within these walls. Rent-a-Center had become an unlikely ally, providing the essentials: a couch that doubled as a guest bed, a table where one could eat or strategize over bills, and a bed that promised rest without the echo of reveille.

My mother, Elaine, had been both proud and a little saddened by my rapid transition. She'd imagined home-cooked meals and late-night tales of European escapades, but independence was a siren song I couldn't ignore—not when every moment as a civilian felt like borrowed time. "I'll visit, Ma," I promised, "and we'll have those talks." But she knew as I did that the boy who left for basic training years ago had returned a man shaped by service and survival.

And then there was her—Mary. Life has a peculiar way of surprising you, and she was a surprise that snuck in unannounced. We met amid the bustling corridors of the very place I now guarded, her laughter a melody that played counterpoint to the monotone existence I had known. It wasn't long before our solitary paths merged into a shared journey.

My life as a civilian had truly begun. Not with fanfare or grand gestures but with small, definitive steps forward. A job to sustain me, a roof to shelter me, and companionship to remind me that there was warmth beyond the cold confines of duty.

As I unpacked the last of my duffel bags, the weight of my medals and ribbons seemed to lighten. They belonged to a chapter that was closing, making way for a narrative still unwritten. The threads of resilience, hope, and perhaps a touch of serendipity were weaving themselves into the fabric of this new life—my life—as I stood ready to meet it head-on.

Fingers stained with ink, I turned the page of the local newspaper, its crinkly texture familiar and somehow comforting. The "Help Wanted" section had become a part of my daily routine—a beacon of possibility in the otherwise mundane existence of my new civilian life. The security guard gig was a paycheck, nothing more. My aspirations climbed higher than the walls of that shopping mall, and each day, I felt an urgency to escape the gravitational pull of minimum wage.

Then, amid the black-and-white clutter of job listings and classifieds, it caught my eye—an ad that seemed almost too good to be true. "Earn $500 a week PLUS commission selling life insurance! No experience required!" The numbers leaped off the page, bold and inviting, promising relief from the financial tightrope I'd been walking since shedding my military uniform.

Life insurance. It was something so mundanely civilian, so far removed from the covert operations and heavy responsibilities of my past life. Yet it beckoned. Five hundred dollars a week—it wasn't just money, it was freedom. Freedom from counting pennies, freedom to dream of a future unshackled by debt and doubt.

I hesitated for just a moment, the formidable doors of my old COMSEC bunker flashing in my mind's eye. I'd safeguarded secrets, codes that could unleash unspeakable power. Now here I was, considering a career peddling peace of mind in paper policies. But resilience is about adaptation, about seizing opportunity when it knocks—or in my case when it's printed between ads for used furniture and part-time waitstaff.

The decision made, I took a deep breath, feeling hope flutter in my chest like a caged bird sensing the sky. With determination, I set out to conquer this new challenge, trading my tactical boots for dress shoes that clicked assertively on the pavement.

In no time at all, I found myself thriving in the world of finance. Selling life insurance wasn't just about persuasion; it was about trust, about being the steadfast rock in a sea of uncertainties. Clients looked into my eyes, searching for honesty, and they found it. They saw someone who knew what it meant to serve, to protect. My military bearing, my unwavering commitment to duty, became my greatest assets in this new theater of operations.

Recognition came swiftly. The accolades of Honor Club agent were pinned to my chest, not unlike the medals of my former life. Yet as I stood among the best of the best, a quiet realization dawned upon me—there was a vast ocean of finance beyond the shores of insurance. My ambition, kindled by the spark of early success, yearned for broader horizons.

As I started flipping through industry magazines instead of newspapers, my thoughts often wandered back to the disciplined chaos of Fort Benning, the heat, the camaraderie, the secret thrill of jumping out of planes. Each memory was a steppingstone, a lesson in courage, adaptability, and the sheer force of will.

"Fortune favors the bold," I mused, the words echoing the sentiments of my drill sergeant from years ago. He was right, of course. Life was not a spectator sport, and I was no longer content to sit on the sidelines.

My path was clear, and although I didn't know it then, this was just the beginning of a journey that would test my mettle in ways the army never did. But for now, I basked in the glow of newfound success, the resilient thread of my past weaving steadily into the hopeful tapestry of my future.

The ring on Mary's finger glinted like a beacon of the future we were supposed to have together. It was a modest thing, much like our dreams: simple yet filled with promise. When she told me about the pregnancy, my heart swelled with a curious mixture of fear and excitement. Fear because doctors had once said I might never be able to father children, and excitement at the prospect of proving them wrong. I loved Mary, despite the whirlwind nature of our relationship, and the thought of starting a family with her, no matter how unexpected, seemed like destiny's hand at play.

But destiny, it seems, is often laced with thorns. Mary's decision to terminate the pregnancy cut through me, her words about dishonor and expectations echoing in the hollow space where anticipation once lived. I could see the strain in her eyes, the way they avoided mine as she spoke of her parents and their community. Even then, a small voice whispered that there was more to her decision than she admitted, but I buried that suspicion beneath layers of trust and hope for our future.

"Life," I reminded myself, "is not about what happens to you but how you respond to it." The resilience I had honed in the military steadied my spirit. And just as one dream began to fade, another beckoned from the pages of the classifieds, an ad that seemed to speak directly to the ambitious flame within me.

"Financial Planner Wanted," it read, and something akin to fate nudged me forward. The interviews came and went, each a stepping stone toward a destiny I hadn't even known to wish for. It was during the final interview, sitting across from the man who held the franchise rights for Northern Ohio, that life threw its next curveball.

"Initially," he said, his voice carrying the weight of consideration, "we saw you fitting into one of our existing offices. But there's something about you—your drive, your background—that makes us think bigger."

Bigger. The word resonated in the room, thrumming with opportunity and challenge. Me running my own office? The thought sent a shiver of exhilaration down my spine. I had always been a soldier, a guardian of secrets and codes, and now I was being handed a new kind of responsibility, one that required a different form of courage.

Life is a series of calculated risks, I mused, my past self-muttering encouragements for the road ahead. I didn't know the first thing about running an office or building a clientele from scratch, but wasn't that the point? To stretch beyond the familiar? To grow in ways I couldn't while standing still?

I left the interview with a sense of purpose that eclipsed the uncertainty clouding my personal life. With every step away from that office, I felt the ground of my new path solidify underfoot. The road wouldn't be easy—I knew that much. But every lesson learned, every trial faced, had prepared me for this.

Fortune favors the bold, echoed in my head, a mantra for the journey ahead. Resilience had brought me this far; hope would carry me further. And luck? Well, luck was simply opportunity meeting preparation. I was ready.

The hinges creaked slightly as I pushed open the door to my future. The office space, now mine, was awash with the cold, early morning light that seemed to hold its breath for a new beginning. There I stood, twenty-three years old and as green as spring's first leaves, yet burning with the fire of ambition. My fingers trembled ever so slightly around the brass of the key, a talisman of the responsibility I'd just shouldered.

"All right, Bobby," I whispered to myself, the sound of my own voice oddly reassuring in the empty room. "This is it."

Craig's proposal had sent my mind into a tailspin—wasn't I too young, too inexperienced to helm such an endeavor? Yet here I was, the paint on the sign that bore my name still fresh, the scent lingering like a promise in the air.

I didn't have much—a few savings bonds from birthdays past, my mother's hesitant optimism, and the gritty determination that had been my most faithful companion since childhood. We three made an unlikely alliance against the world of finance that sprawled out before me, uncharted and daunting.

"Fortune favors the bold," I reminded myself, feeling the weight of the phrase settle in my chest. The military's shadow still haunted the corners of my life, but here, in this nascent sanctuary of dreams, I was free to shape my destiny.

One foot in front of the other, I moved through the space, my hands ghosting over surfaces that would soon thrum with the energy of business. The used furniture was a mishmash of styles and eras—each piece a silent witness to someone else's history, ready to be part of mine.

With the phone cradled between shoulder and ear, I dialed numbers at random, the white pages open like a roadmap to potential futures. Each ring was a heartbeat, each voicemail a deferral of judgment, but I persisted. This was the grind, the hustle—the call to arms for every dreamer who dared.

"Hi, this is Bobby Quayle, your local financial planner. May I have a moment of your time to discuss how we can secure your financial future?"

The words felt foreign at first, but with repetition, they became a mantra, shaping the reality I yearned to create.

When not on the phone, I walked among my community, shaking hands with local businessmen and women at Chamber of Commerce meetings, sharing Rotary lunches, and discussing community projects with Kiwanis members. With each handshake, I sowed seeds of trust, and with each smile, I watered the soil of opportunity.

As dusk crept in, painting the sky with the colors of closing day, the office remained dark and quiet. But the silence no longer felt empty—it hummed with the echoes of potential connections, the whispers of deals yet to be struck, and the soft murmur of hope that refused to be quelled.

"Tomorrow," I said, locking the door behind me, the key cool and solid in my grasp, "we go again."

Hope sprouted within me, tenacious and wild, and I nurtured it with thoughts of what could be. The path ahead was fogged with uncertainty, but I had weathered storms before. Resilience was etched into the very marrow of my bones. Tomorrow, indeed, was another chance to prove it.

CHAPTER 11

GREAT SUCCESS AND EVEN GREATER BETRAYALS

The steady hum of voices and the clatter of calculators served as a symphony to my aspirations, a testament to the frantic pace at which my life had transformed. The office, once barren and echoing with the silence of uncertainty, now thrived with the energy of ambition and enterprise. My desk was a command center, littered with financial statements and business plans, while the CPA I had partnered with, a meticulous man with a hawk's eye for numbers, occupied the adjacent room.

"Another good quarter," he'd say, handing over reports that reflected our mutual success. Our collaboration flourished; his clients became mine and mine his. Together, we fortified financial futures.

Thursdays brought a new rhythm to the office as the estate planning attorney would stroll in with her leather-bound briefcase, ready to dispense advice to those seeking to safeguard their legacies. Her presence was both a beacon of wisdom and a bridge to another vital aspect of the financial services we provided. Clients left our meetings with more than just reassurance—they left with a plan stitched into the fabric of their lives.

In the midst of it all, I found myself standing before my peers at the Chamber of Commerce, the weight of the president's gavel comfortable in my hand. It wasn't just the title that mattered—it was the recognition, the affirmation that my voice carried weight, that my ideas could shape the community I had come to cherish.

But beneath the surface of this burgeoning success lay a gnawing unease, a whisper of discord that crept into my consciousness during the quiet hours. Small discrepancies in paperwork, evasive answers to direct questions, laughter that didn't quite reach the eyes—my partners' actions slowly painted a picture that didn't match the one I held in my head.

I wrestled with the discomfort, pushing it aside, convincing myself that it was nothing more than the usual bumps in any business venture. But the seed of doubt, once planted, refused to be ignored. A year rolled by, each day tainted by the growing suspicion that my trust was misplaced, that the foundation I stood upon was built on sand.

It took time to accept what my gut had known all along. With every fiber of my being resisting, I conceded to the truth—the camaraderie I thought existed was merely a facade. My partners, though adept at playing their parts, harbored intentions that did not align with mine. The realization stung, an unpleasant echo of past betrayals.

So with the lessons of the past heavy on my shoulders, I made the difficult decision to disentangle myself from the partnership. In a move that felt like cutting off a limb to save the body, I sold my interests, severing ties that had become more shackle than support.

Yet even as I stepped away from what I had built, fate extended a new opportunity. A national bank sought a branch manager, and my experience had not gone unnoticed. Interviews led to offers, and offers led to decisions that promised a fresh start.

As I stood at the precipice of this next chapter, I couldn't help but marvel at the journey. From the military to finance, from a novice to a leader, each step was a building block, each setback a lesson in disguise. The office may have been quieter now, absent the buzz of shared ambition, but within its walls echoed the indomitable spirit of hope and the unwavering resolve to forge ahead.

"Resilience," I whispered to the empty room, a promise and a proclamation. "We go again."

Staring out the window of my soon-to-be former office, a reflection caught my eye—it was a distorted image of myself, and in it, I saw the weight of recent revelations pulling at the corners of my resolve. The sky outside mirrored my internal turmoil, clouds heavy with unshed rain, threatening to break at any moment.

As I packed the last of my personal effects into a cardboard box, the weight of the past felt tangible in my hands. The framed photo of Mary and me, taken in a time of innocent love, now seemed like a relic from another life. Each item was a piece of the puzzle that was Bobby Quayle, a tableau of triumphs and defeats.

I picked up the old army coin I kept on my desk, running my thumb over its worn edges, remembering the young man I once was, head full of dreams and heart full of courage. That same spirit stirred within me now, urging me to look not at what I had lost but at what remained to be gained.

"Resilience," I whispered again, this time with conviction. I had weathered storms before, and while the horizon ahead was dark with uncertainty, I would navigate through it. I had to.

With the box under my arm and the door closing behind me, I stepped into the corridor, its fluorescent lights flickering a stark goodbye. The future awaited, unwritten and untamed, and I was the author of my own destiny. This was not an end but a beginning. A promise that no matter how fierce the tempest, there was always a chance to rebuild, to find new land beyond the wreckage.

"Hope," I said aloud as I made my way to the exit. The word echoed off the walls, a mantra for the journey ahead. "We go again."

My marriage, once a safe haven, had become a stormy sea of deceit. I'd noticed the signs: the late nights Mary claimed were spent with friends or working late, the strange numbers on the phone bill, the scent of unfamiliar cologne lingering on her clothes. It wasn't just intuition anymore; it was an agonizing awareness that crept into my bones and settled there. With each passing day, the evidence mounted, and so did my sense of betrayal.

And then, like a bolt from the blue, came the news about my ex-partner. My television buzzed with the headline: "Local Financial Planner Indicted for Fraud"—and his face, a portrait of greed I thought I'd left behind, splashed across the screen. Over $8 million stolen from those who had trusted us, trusted me by association. A sickening knot tightened in my stomach as I read on. Before he could be brought to justice, before he could face the consequences of his choices, he had made the most final decision of all—a gunshot, a life ended, and with it any chance for answers or closure.

I leaned back in my chair, the leather creaking beneath me. Part of me wanted to rage against the injustice, to scream at the universe for stacking the deck so unfairly. But deep down, I knew this was yet another trial to endure, another test of the resilience that had been both my armor and my curse.

"Challenges," I muttered to the empty room, the word tasting bitter on my tongue. And yet a flicker of hope ignited within me. They say luck favors the prepared, and if life had taught me anything, it was to remain ever vigilant, ever ready to adapt.

CHAPTER 12

You Can't Do That!

The courthouse doors swung shut behind me with a finality that felt like the closing of an era. Mary, in her characteristic assertive stride, walked ahead—the short Greek woman with the loud voice whom I had once vowed to cherish. Now all she took with her was the house, leaving me with a mountain of debt wrapped around my shoulders like a lead cloak. It wasn't fair; it never is in love and war. But this... this was the quickest route to peace, to silence the clamor of a fractured marriage.

I stood for a moment, watching her disappear down the marble corridor, the echo of her footsteps mingling with the muffled sounds of justice being doled out behind oak doors. My mind wandered to the movie hero Rocky Balboa, his words about life's harsh realities resonating within me. Yeah, life could indeed be mean and nasty.

Later, slumped in the leather chair across from my attorney, the weight of Rocky's truth pressed even heavier. The room smelled of old books and worn-in wood, and the attorney, a man of sharp eyes and tailored suits, laid out my options like cards on the table.

"Bankruptcy, Bobby," he said with a sigh, "it's your best bet."

"Although you dissolved your relationship with the partners and none of your clients were affected, creditors and his victims could still try to come after you. Guilt by previous association, so to speak." His words stung, but they carried a note of truth that was hard to ignore.

So nodding silently, I consented to the path set before me—bankruptcy. It was a bitter pill, yet I couldn't help but feel a sense of liberation. Walking away from two dishonest partners, severing the bonds with a toxic past, I held on to hope and the belief that sometimes you need to be stripped bare to begin anew.

"Life ain't all sunshine and rainbows," I murmured to myself as I signed the documents, the pen scratching loudly in the quiet room. The phrase became a mantra, a grounding reminder that I was no stranger to adversity. My reflection in the window showed a man changed by life's battles, brown hair cropped short out of practicality rather than style, and eyes that had seen too much yet still looked forward with resilience.

"Thank you," I said to the attorney, my voice steady, betraying none of the storm inside. He gave me a curt nod, understanding perhaps that this was more than just a legal procedure for me. It was a cleansing fire, burning away the remnants of a life I was ready to leave behind.

As I stepped out into the sunlight, the world didn't look any different, but I did. Bankrupt in finance, perhaps, but not in spirit. I had weathered worse, and I would rise again. The road ahead was uncertain, paved with challenges and devoid of shortcuts, but I had always been good at finding my way through the wilderness.

"Adapt and overcome," I told myself. There was hope in the journey, luck to be found in the most unexpected places, and strength in the belief that no matter how hard the hit, moving forward was the only way to win. And win I would.

The night air felt different, almost electric, as I slid into the driver's seat of my red Pontiac Grand Am—the one thing I had managed to keep through the bankruptcy. The leather hugged my body, a familiar comfort amid the chaos that had been my life recently. I inhaled deeply, the new car smell mingling with a sense of freedom that sparked within me. It was a celebration, an opportunity to embrace the end of one chapter and the start of another. I was dressed sharp, feeling confident, perhaps even a little reckless. I wanted to taste life again, feel its rhythms, its unpredictable nature.

I found myself at a club called the Bomber's Squadron, with neon lights pulsing like the heartbeat of the night. The music vibrated through the walls, a siren's call luring me inside. There, amid the laughter and clinking glasses, I met her—a woman with a smile that promised adventure. We danced, we drank, we lost ourselves in conversation. As the hours passed, the connection between us grew undeniable. When she suggested we head back to her place, I didn't hesitate.

The spell of the evening was intoxicating. Everything felt heightened, vivid, alive. But as dawn approached, reality started to seep back in. She offered me a ride back to the club where my car awaited, her kindness a gentle reminder of the goodness that still existed in the world. Stepping out onto the parking lot, however, delivered a brutal jolt. Where my Pontiac should have been, there was nothing but empty space. Stolen. My heart sank, a heavy anchor pulling down the fleeting joy of the past hours.

"Are you sure this is where you parked?" Her voice was tinged with concern, but I hardly heard her. My mind raced—divorce, bankruptcy, and now this? A cruel joke played by fate, no doubt. The insurance company's response was just as merciless. "Fair market" value, they said, a figure that fell laughably short of the loan I still owed. Fair for who? Certainly not for me.

There, in the early morning light, I stood on the precipice of despair. Yet within me, a flicker of something unbreakable stirred. I wouldn't let this break me. Life had thrown punches before, and each time I had found the strength to rise, to adapt, to move forward. This would be no different. I had survived the tempest of divorce, navigated the murky waters of bankruptcy, and I would find a way to overcome this too.

"Thanks for the ride," I told her as she dropped me off at my apartment, forcing a smile. "I'll figure this out." She nodded, offering a sympathetic look before driving away. Alone, I watched the sunrise paint the sky in shades of hope—a canvas of possibility. This was just another test, another chance to prove my resilience. And as the first rays of sunlight touched my face, I knew deep down that luck hadn't abandoned me; it was simply waiting for me to seize it once again.

Stepping onto the first of three buses, my breath materialized before me in the chill of predawn, a ghostly testament to the change in my fortunes. The once familiar comfort of leather and the hum of an engine had been traded for the staccato rhythm of a transit ride—three transfers, each a link in the chain that bound me to a routine I hadn't chosen but fiercely owned.

"Adapt and overcome, Bobby," whispered the gritty voice of resilience within me, the echo of an old Army buddy's mantra blending seamlessly with Rocky's cinematic creed. It was a battle cry against the odds, a refusal to yield to life's low blows.

I grasped the cold metal pole as the bus lurched into motion, the city beginning to stir outside the fogged windows. Each stop a reminder of the miles between where I was and where I needed to be. The journey was long, nearly two hours spent navigating the early morning sprawl that could have been traversed in a fraction of the time by car. Yet there was something almost meditative about it, a forced pause that allowed me to reflect, plan, and steel myself for the day ahead.

Each jolt of the bus served as a physical manifestation of the setbacks I'd endured—divorce, debt, the disappearance of what little I'd managed to hold on to. But I wasn't one to dwell on misfortune. Instead, I saw each day's commute as a small victory, a testament to my tenacity.

"Next stop: Elm Street," droned the robotic voice of the bus intercom, snapping me back to reality. With each transfer, I grew more determined, feeling the grind of this new reality like grit under my fingernails. It was gritty, yes, but not insurmountable. Not for me.

The hours added up, time I could have spent sleeping or working, yet also time that proved my resolve. I watched the revolving cast of fellow commuters, each absorbed in their own silent battles. We were all warriors in the trenches of daily life, armed with briefcases or backpacks instead of rifles.

By the last leg of the trip, the sun would peek over the horizon, casting long shadows and bathing the world in a golden hue. Hope rode alongside me, whispering promises of a future unburdened by debt, a future where I could reclaim some measure of control.

For now, my ledger remained in the red, the car loan a persistent anchor. But with each paycheck from the banking job, I chipped away at the balance, saving diligently for the day when I could sit behind the wheel of a car that was truly mine again.

"Adversity introduces a man to himself," they say, and through these trials, I was becoming well-acquainted with the man I was and the man I was still becoming. Resilient. Resourceful. Unyielding.

The bus pulled into the stop nearest to the bank, and as I stepped off, I straightened my tie—my armor against the world—and walked toward the glass doors with purpose. Inside, numbers awaited, figures to be tallied and accounts to be balanced. Life, too, was a ledger, and I was determined to make mine balance out in the end.

For every setback, there was a comeback waiting to be written. And as the doors slid open, welcoming me into the cool air of the lobby, I carried with me the unwavering belief that luck had not deserted me—it was simply biding its time, ready for the moment when I seized it with both hands.

I slip into the driver's seat of my new car, a tangible symbol of perseverance and triumph. The scent of fresh leather mingles with the crisp autumn air, serving as a reminder of the journey that brought me here—a testament to the resilience that has carried me through life's gauntlet. As I turn the key, the engine hums to life, and I feel a surge of pride. This isn't just a new car; it's the fruit of six months of frugality, of early mornings waiting on cold bus benches, of relentless determination.

The drive to the bank is smooth, the roads familiar. Every pothole and stop sign is a memory from my youth, each turn taking me closer to a place that holds my history in its walls. It's surreal to think that this building, where I once made my first deposit from a summer job, is now under my stewardship. My hands grip the wheel tighter at the thought. Hometown boy makes good—the local narrative writes itself.

The day Shelly walked into the bank, her presence was like a beacon cutting through the monotonous sea of numbers and transactions. She had this air about her—regal yet approachable—that drew my eyes from the spreadsheets on my monitor to her figure silhouetted against the sunlit entrance. Initially, she was just another client with a problem that needed solving, but as I guided her through the financial maze, I couldn't help noticing the way her brow furrowed in concentration, the graceful movement of her pen as she took notes.

After ensuring her immediate concerns were addressed, I found myself taking a leap—something inside urged me to ask her out. It wasn't impulsive; it felt right, like stepping forward when every sense tells you there's solid ground ahead. We dated for over a year, our conversations a blend of her measured tones and my frank, soldierly speak. I never did understand the power words held over her, how *fuck* could be a grenade and *shit* a landmine. To me, they were nothing more than vocal punctuation, marks of emphasis in the story I narrated daily.

Shelly and I, we were an unlikely pairing—different temperaments, different tastes, different ways of seeing the world. Yet somehow, we clicked. They say opposites attract, and we were living proof. Our union was a dance of nearly two decades, a choreography that saw us glide and stumble through life's unpredictable rhythms. The challenging times we were yet to face in the army and a business we ventured into together later was both our stage and our storm, and when it collapsed, so did the fragile bridge connecting our disparate worlds.

As I reflect on those years now, I see them not as wasted time but as chapters rich with learning, moments steeped in the essence of life. Our relationship may have ended, but the legacy of our trials lingers—a testament to my belief that every experience, good or bad, contributes a verse to the epic poem of one's existence.

Standing here in the bank where it all began, amid the hum of machines and quiet chatter of patrons, I'm reminded that life is a mosaic of such encounters. Each person we meet adds a tile, a splash of color to the grand design. And while the pattern might seem chaotic at times, there is beauty in the complexity, hope in the fragments.

I turn away from the counter, feeling the weight of the past but buoyed by the knowledge that resilience has been my faithful companion through it all. It's not just about weathering the storm but also dancing in the rain, finding joy in the midst of adversity.

Luck hasn't abandoned me; it's woven into the fabric of my being, threaded through my narrative like gold through granite.

So as I prepare to close up my till and step into the evening's embrace, I carry with me an introspective hope. The sun will set, the night will fall, but come morning, the horizon will glow with the promise of a new day—a canvas awaiting the bold strokes of continued determination and the subtle hues of hard-won wisdom.

Inside the bank, the quiet buzz of productivity is a symphony to my ears. I watch as customers interact with tellers, their lives intersecting with ours for brief, transactional moments. It's here, in these exchanges, that I found my calling, not just in numbers and accounts but in understanding people, in securing their futures.

My office door closes behind me with a soft click, and I take a moment to survey my domain—awards line the shelves, including the crystal plaque celebrating our branch's achievement in loan volume. On another, a golden statuette stands proudly, recognition of my success in annuity sales. They are not just accolades but mile markers on a long road traveled.

The phone rings, snapping me back to the present. The voice on the other end congratulates me, extending an invitation to speak in Las Vegas as a keynote speaker on financial planning and annuity sales. I accept with a humble thanks, feeling the weight of the opportunity. To share my insights, to guide others on paths of prosperity—it's more than an honor; it's a service.

As I hang up the phone, my gaze drifts to the window, watching the world go by. The leaves have turned, gold and crimson dancing in the wind, a visual echo of change, of cycles, of rebirth. Life has thrown me punches, some that left bruises, but none that could keep me down. I've learned to roll with them, to stand back up, to adapt.

Hope has been the steadfast drumbeat pushing me forward, the belief that no matter how dire the circumstances, there's a chance for redemption, for glory. You see, luck isn't just chance; it's the result of hard work meeting opportunity. And maybe there's something in the soil of this town that nurtures such fortitude—I'd like to think so.

My reflection in the glass stares back at me, a man molded by trials, shaped by victories. It whispers of potential yet untapped, of stories yet written. There's an entire horizon out there, painted with the hues of possibility, and I am ready to chase the sunrise.

As dusk settles over the town, I lock up the branch, the day's successes and challenges neatly filed away. Stepping out into the cooling evening, I look up at the sky, where the first stars are beginning to twinkle. They remind me that even in darkness, there is light to be found, guidance to be sought.

Life, in all its unpredictable glory, moves with the certainty of time. And I move with it, ever hopeful, forever resilient, my heart beating in time with the unyielding rhythm of progress and the unwavering faith in tomorrow's luck.

With each morning that dawned, I found myself tracing the same familiar route to the bank, my hands automatically following the rituals of unlocking doors, disarming alarms, and powering up systems. These motions had become second nature, a dance of digits and keys that had charted my course for two decades.

But this morning was different. The air held a stillness, a hush before the storm. As I stepped into my office, the phone rang with a call that would redraw the map of my life. "Bobby, it's about the merger," George Mitchell's voice came through the line, a harbinger of the chaos unraveling in the financial world. It was 2008 and banks were folding like houses of cards. "We're downsizing. I'm sorry, but your position is no longer available."

The words hit like a gut punch, stealing the breath from my lungs. In the span of a heartbeat, twenty years of climbing, of striving and achieving, seemed to crumble into dust. The bank was closing. My bank was closing. And with it, a chapter of my life was forcibly concluded.

Shelly sat across from me at our modest kitchen table that evening, her eyes searching mine for a flicker of hope. "What are we going to do?" she asked, her voice steady despite the tremor of uncertainty that underpinned her words.

I gazed back at her, letting the silence stretch between us as I grappled with the magnitude of our situation. We were at a crossroads, the path behind us eroded by an economic maelstrom, and the road ahead shrouded in fog. The only certainty was the love and trust that bound us together, stronger than any market force.

"Jobs are scarce," I admitted, running a hand through my short-cropped hair. "Especially for someone with my background, in these times." I spread out the classifieds, the pages dotted with far too many "positions filled" and "applications closed." With every turned page, my resolve hardened. "But we'll get through this, Shelly. We always do."

The nights grew longer as I scoured listings and sent out resumes, each one seeming to vanish into the void. Banks were retreating, battening down the hatches, and the few roles available were commission-based gambles that promised more risk than reward.

As Shelly left each day to continue her work as a social worker, a profession mercifully insulated from the financial collapse, I remained at home, surrounded by the quiet walls of our living room. It was there, amid the stacks of job postings and unanswered emails, that the stark reality settled upon me—we could either drain our savings dry or I could forge a new path.

"Perhaps it's time for something new," I murmured to myself, staring out the window where the first leaves of autumn were beginning to turn. "A different journey."

And so I began to look beyond the familiar horizon of finance, considering opportunities I had never imagined. I attended workshops, networked with professionals from various fields, and discovered that my skills were not confined to the world of banking. There were other industries, other roles where a man who understood numbers and people could make a difference. With each passing day, I felt the embers of hope stirring within me. This was not the end, merely a redirection—a chance to reinvent myself, to prove that the resilience which had carried me this far would not falter now. "Adversity," I reminded myself, "is just another word for opportunity."

As dusk fell and Shelly returned home, I shared my thoughts with her, the ideas taking shape like constellations in the night sky. Our conversation meandered through possibilities and dreams, the kindling of a future not yet written. "Whatever happens," I said, looking deep into her eyes, "we'll face it together."

In the quiet of the evening, as the stars emerged above, I found comfort in their silent testimony. They were witnesses to countless stories of struggle and triumph, and now they watched over ours. Our luck hadn't run out; it was simply waiting to be seized once more. And with each twinkling light, I felt the resurgence of a familiar drumbeat—the beat of resilience, of hope, and the undying belief in the fortune that lay just beyond the bend.

The cool evening breeze brushed against my skin as I lounged in the backyard, my gaze following Mandy's energetic pursuit of the squirrels that dared to trespass her domain. The Border Collie mix zigzagged across the lawn, her focus unbreakable. In that simple, carefree moment, inspiration struck me like a bolt from the blue. "I will go back into the army!"

The words tumbled out before I could temper them with doubt, surprising both Shelly and Mandy, who paused mid-chase to consider me with tilted heads.

The idea might have sounded ludicrous even to my own ears, but it carried a weight of conviction that anchored it to reality. "I can get back into shape," I continued, fleshing out the vision, "and go back into the army as an intelligence analyst, then on to Warrant Officer School."

Shelly's skepticism was palpable, as tangible as the fading light that draped over us. "*YOU CAN'T DO THAT!* You're forty-three years old and not in shape. What makes you think that you could get back in at this age? And how would you deal with combat in Afghanistan?" Her concerns were valid. Yet the very act of verbalizing my goal seemed to breathe life into it, lending it substance and energy.

"Age is just a number, Shelly," I responded, my voice steady with burgeoning resolve. "And as for shape—well, that's within my control, isn't it?"

As I spoke, memories of my past challenges drifted through my mind—the divorce, the bankruptcy, and those long hours commuting by bus, each one a testament to my tenacity. I had been beaten down before, but I had always clawed my way back up. The naysayers in my life, those voices of well-intentioned caution, only stoked the fires of my determination. They didn't see the world through my eyes; they didn't feel the burn of ambition in their veins as I did. "The more I'm told I can't do something, the more I want to prove them wrong," I said quietly, almost to myself.

Shelly watched me, her expression softening. She knew me better than anyone—knew that once a seed of possibility was planted in my mind, I would nurture it with relentless dedication until it blossomed into reality.

The sky deepened to a velvety indigo, stars peppering the heavens in silent encouragement. They didn't blink at the immensity of my dream. Instead, they shone steadily, as if to remind me that the universe was vast and full of paths yet to be taken. "Adversity," I mused aloud, "is just another word for opportunity." It was a mantra that had seen me through dark times, a lifeline thrown across tumultuous seas. And now it was a clarion call to action. "Whatever happens," I declared, turning to meet Shelly's gaze, "we'll face it together."

The bond between us was unspoken, an invisible thread woven through our shared history, resilient as spider silk. In the growing stillness of the evening, the night sky bore witness to the resilience that hummed beneath my skin. Luck hadn't abandoned me—it was merely biding its time, waiting for me to reach out and grab hold of it with both hands. And in the quiet certainty of that thought, I found hope flickering anew, ready to guide me toward the next chapter of an unwritten story.

Sweat beaded on my forehead, each drop a testament to the grueling regimen I had committed myself to. The gym's air was thick with determination, mine mingled with that of every other soul pushing their limits within these walls. I pounded the treadmill, the rhythmic thud of my sneakers syncing with the pulsating beats of Rocky's theme song funneling through my earbuds. "It's not about how hard you can hit, it's about how hard you can get hit and keep moving forward," Stallone's gritty voice instructed me. It became a mantra that fueled each stride, each mile. On alternate days, the whirring of a stationary bike filled my ears as I envisioned the open road beneath me, the resistance knob cranked just high enough to mimic an uphill battle. Because that's what this was—a battle against time, against age, against every naysayer who ever doubted the fire still burning in my gut. And then there were the weights, cold and unyielding in my grasp, challenging me to lift a little more than last time, to feel the satisfying burn that told me my body hadn't given up on me yet.

"Hydrate or die," the two former *Biggest Loser* contestants would chant, their own sweat-soaked shirts a badge of honor. They knew the mountain I was scaling; they had faced their own. So I took their advice like scripture, guzzling a gallon of water daily until my system flushed with vitality, until my skin held the glow of a man reborn. In just two months, the mirror reflected not the weary survivor of life's cruel twists but the warrior who had once stood tall in uniform. Nearly fifty pounds shed, a transformation not just of body but of spirit. My old self—the soldier, the fighter—stared back at me with familiar intensity.

We both nodded, acknowledging the readiness that thrummed through my veins. Pushups and sit-ups were now child's play, a prelude to the endurance test I knew awaited me. I could run two miles in a breeze, my lungs no longer begging for mercy but hungry for the challenge. They say luck is the residue of design. Well, I had designed this comeback meticulously, with the hope that had never truly left me, even when the shadows loomed close. Now as I geared up for the fitness test that would seal my fate, I felt that same hope wrap around me like a cloak, insulating me from doubt. "Adversity is just another word for opportunity," I reminded myself, the mantra merging with the symphony of exertion around me. Each step forward was a march toward destiny, each breath a whisper of potential.

There were no guarantees, no crystal ball to show me where this path would lead. But in this moment, soaked in sweat and the sweet satisfaction of progress, I was certain of one thing: the only luck I needed was the kind forged from my own resilience. And in that, I was already rich beyond measure. The morning sun was just cresting the horizon as I stepped onto the training grounds of Fort Sill, Oklahoma. A crisp breeze brushed against my face, carrying with it the scents of dew-soaked grass and the distant musk of the firing range. Today was the day—the physical fitness test that would mark my return to the army after nearly two decades. My heart thrummed in my chest, not from nerves but from a wellspring of hope that had been steadily filling me, drop by drop, throughout my intense months of training.

I eyed the obstacle course ahead, a serpentine path of challenges designed to push soldiers to their limits. Each station stood as a testament to the resilience demanded of the men and women who served, and now, as I laced up my boots with hands steady and sure, I felt a kinship with these silent sentinels of fortitude. "Let's see what you've got, Quayle," I muttered to myself, a half-grin creeping across my face. The words weren't just a challenge; they were an affirmation.

The crunch of gravel underfoot became my drumbeat as I approached the starting line, each step a declaration that I was back—not just in body but in spirit. As the whistle pierced the air, signaling the start of the test, I launched forward. Pushups and sit-ups, once my adversaries, now felt like old friends greeting me with open arms. The rhythm of exertion was cathartic, a symphony of strength played out on the canvas of my muscles. With each rep, I shed the weight of doubt, my body moving with the precision of a well-oiled machine.

Then came the range, the familiar scent of gunpowder wafting through the air like an old cologne. The rifle nestled into my shoulder as if it had never left, an extension of my own will. One shot after another rang out, each finding its mark with the confidence of years etched into muscle memory. Watching the targets topple felt like knocking down the barriers of age and expectation, one bullet at a time.

But it was the Combat Lifesavers course that truly tested the mettle I had forged in the fires of adversity. There, surrounded by my peers, I learned to bring calm to chaos. The intimacy of saving a life, even in practice, was profound. As I applied tourniquets and slid IV needles into willing veins, a sense of purpose swelled within me. This wasn't just about proving I could come back; it was about being ready to stand shoulder to shoulder with those who might one day depend on me.

Breathless and drenched in sweat, I finished the day with a feeling that transcended exhaustion. It was a cocktail of triumph and humility, knowing that I had not only met the standard but soared above it. The youthful faces around me, some awash with awe, others with respect, told me all I needed to know.

"Quayle, looks like you've still got it," one of the instructors remarked, offering a quick, approving nod.

"Still got it? Sir, I never lost it," I replied, allowing myself the luxury of a broad smile. But there was truth in jest—I might have been bent by life's harsh lessons, but I was far from broken.

As dusk settled over Fort Sill, painting the sky in shades of purple and gold, I stood alone for a moment, reflecting on the journey that had brought me here. The road had been long, fraught with pitfalls and pain, but also paved with persistence and hope.

"*Adversity* is just another word for opportunity," I whispered to the falling night, the mantra that had become my lodestar. In the quiet of the evening, with stars beginning to twinkle into existence, I knew that luck hadn't carried me to this point—it was something much more potent.

Resilience. Hope. And the unwavering belief that no matter how many times life knocks you down, there's always a chance to rise, to fight, to soar. That was the real secret, the truest form of luck anyone could ever hold. And as I turned toward the barracks, I carried that secret with me, a talisman against whatever tomorrow might bring.

The first rays of morning light spilled across the desert landscape, casting long shadows from the barracks that had become my temporary home at Fort Huachuca. The crisp Arizona air felt like a new beginning as I laced up my boots and prepared for another day reacquainting myself with military life. The world had evolved since I last wore the uniform, and nowhere was this more evident than in the technology that now underpinned modern intelligence operations.

In the classrooms and labs where youthful soldiers eagerly absorbed information, I found myself a student once again. Lines of code replaced field notes; satellites tracked where once we only had maps. I adjusted my mindset, allowed myself to be molded by this new era of warfare. It wasn't just about learning; it was about adapting, embracing the fluidity of change. My resolve did not waver, despite the occasional feeling of being a relic in a digital age.

Between sessions, I found sanctuary in the pages of textbooks for the college course I had enrolled in. A degree in intelligence operations wasn't just another accolade; it represented a bridge to my future, a testament to the fact that growth and learning do not recognize age or circumstance.

When the time came to leave Fort Huachuca's structured environment just six months later, I packed my duffel bag with a sense of accomplishment. The threads of knowledge I'd gathered were woven into a tapestry of renewed purpose. I was ready for my next assignment, but more than that, I was eager to reunite with Shelly and Mandy. Distance had only deepened my appreciation for them, turning thoughts of reunion into a beacon that guided me through the most demanding days.

Arriving in El Paso, the reality of our situation settled in like the dust kicked up by desert winds. Housing on base was an elusive dream, reserved for those who had the luxury of time. I didn't. With the pragmatism that had seen me through darker days, I scoured the city and secured a modest house in a quiet suburb—our new haven amid uncertainty.

I busied myself with making the place feel like home. A coat of fresh paint here, some minor repairs there; each stroke of the brush felt like a declaration of resilience. This was more than refurbishing a building; it was laying down roots for the next chapter of our lives.

The day I flew back to Ohio to help with the move, anticipation thrummed through my veins. Standing at the doorstep, suitcase in hand, I could hardly contain my excitement. Mandy's joyful barking greeted me before I even turned the key in the lock, her tail wagging furiously as she leapt into my arms. In her eyes, there was no reproach for my absence, only boundless love and an eagerness for what lay ahead. It struck me then that hope is often reflected best in the eyes of those who wait for us, unwavering in their faith.

As I loaded our belongings into the moving truck, I realized that every box, every piece of furniture, was infused with memories of struggle and triumph. They weren't just possessions; they were fragments of a life lived authentically, fearlessly. And as we began our journey toward El Paso, I carried with me not just the tangible pieces of our past but also an unshakable hope for the future.

"*Adversity* is just another word for opportunity," I reminded myself, the mantra echoing in my heart with each mile we covered. Life had indeed knocked me down, more times than I cared to count. But each time, I had risen, driven by the belief that luck isn't something you find. It's something you create through grit, through grace, and through an indomitable will to keep moving forward.

The morning sun cast a warm glow over the familiar bricks of our Ohio home as I pulled the last of our suitcases down the porch steps. Shelly was inside, saying her farewells to the house that had sheltered us through so many seasons of life. I could hear the muffled sound of her voice laced with nostalgia as she walked from room to room, her footsteps a soft echo against hardwood floors worn smooth by time.

I turned to face the neighborhood, its lawns speckled with dew and the chorus of birdsong punctuating the silence of departure. We had become fixtures here, woven into the tapestry of community barbecues, borrowed tools, and shared triumphs. But as much as this place was a tapestry, it was also a cocoon—one we were now ready to shed.

"Goodbye, Bobby." Mrs. Peterson, from next door, clasped my hand between hers, her eyes moist but her smile unwavering. "You take care of yourself out there."

"Will do, Mrs. Peterson," I replied, squeezing her hands gently. "And thank you for everything."

We exchanged no more words, just a knowing nod—a mutual understanding that well-wishes were also silent prayers for safekeeping.

Turning my back on the life we knew was akin to stepping off a cliff, trusting that the parachute of hope would unfurl in time. It was an act of faith, a belief in the possibility that lay beyond the horizon. Yet as I looked at the moving truck, its belly full of the remnants of yesterday, a sense of purpose steadied my resolve.

"Ready?" Shelly's voice broke through my reverie, her presence beside me sudden but welcome.

"More than ever," I said, offering her a smile that carried the weight of our collective courage.

With one last glance, I climbed into the cab of the truck, the engine roaring to life beneath me. We were leaving behind walls that had absorbed laughter and witnessed tears, but we were taking with us the strength they had given us—the resilience that had been forged within their confines.

As we pulled away, the rearview mirror framed the shrinking image of our old home, now entrusted to strangers who would build their own stories within its embrace. Life, in its relentless march forward, waits for no one, but it also offers the chance to redefine oneself with each new dawn.

Our journey to El Paso was not just a relocation; it was a pilgrimage toward the promise of reinvention. The road unfurled ahead, a ribbon of asphalt symbolizing the continuity of our narrative. There would be challenges, certainly—there always are—but the anticipation of growth made every mile a testament to human potential.

"Here's to new beginnings," Shelly said, her voice steady and sure.

"Here's to creating our own luck," I added, feeling the truth of those words resonate deep within.

The future was unwritten, a blank page on which we would inscribe the next chapter of our lives. And I knew, with a certainty that bordered on prophecy, that the story ahead was ours to tell—ours to live—with all the tenacity and optimism we could muster.

Adversity had indeed been my tutor, teaching me lessons I never sought but always valued. Now, as we drove into the heart of a new adventure, I was reminded that life is not about avoiding the storms but about learning to dance in the rain, embracing each drop as a harbinger of the harvest to come.

CHAPTER 13

MY CAREER IN THE ARMY 2.0

The U-Haul rumbled along the interstate like a steadfast mule, carrying our lives in its belly. I was at the helm, my hands gripping the wheel with a sense of purpose only the prospect of a new beginning can instill. Behind me, Shelly followed faithfully in her Prius, Mandy, our loyal border collie mix, riding shotgun, her nose pressed to the window as she took in the ever-changing landscape.

Every couple of hours, we'd pull over at some rest stop or gas station, stretching our legs and letting Mandy scamper around to burn off her cooped-up energy. Each time I stepped down from the truck, a sharp reminder would shoot up my spine—a relentless ache that had been my unwelcome companion since Fort Sill.

The combative training there had been tough, and meant to push us to our limits. It was a dance of technique and endurance, but it wasn't the kind of pain that comes with muscle growth—it was deeper, more insidious. The kind that gnaws at you when you're trying to sleep or when you're miles into a long drive to a place like El Paso. But pain is a funny thing; it has a way of teaching you about your own resilience. With every throb, I was reminded that I've been through worse, seen darker days, and still emerged with my head held high. My back may have ached, but my spirit remained unbroken.

"Everything okay, Bobby?" Shelly's voice crackled through the car window on one of our stops, her eyes filled with concern.

"Nothing I can't handle," I replied with a half-grin, not wanting to worry her more than necessary. "Just the usual aches."

"Take it easy. Remember, it's not a race," she soothed, Mandy's head popping up behind her as if to echo the sentiment.

"Never is," I assured her and meant it. I've learned patience the hard way—by having none and paying the price.

As we got closer to El Paso, the ache in my back seemed to crescendo, each mile marker a drumbeat to which my body resonated. Still, I kept driving, my mind focused not on the discomfort but on the hope and promise that lay ahead.

El Paso was more than just our destination; it was a symbol of progress, of moving forward despite the challenges. And as the city's lights began to twinkle in the distance, a sense of accomplishment settled over me. It might have taken two and a half days, countless breaks, and a good deal of gritting my teeth against the pain, but we had made it.

And if history has taught me anything, it's that the journey is just as important as the destination. So I'd take the aching back, the weary muscles, and the endless highway because they were all part of the story—a story of never giving in, no matter what life throws your way.

As we continued our trek to El Paso, memories of that day at Fort Sill crept their way into my thoughts. Gritting my teeth, I squared off with the ex-Marine across the matted floor of Fort Sill's combative training room. He was a mountain of a man, a good two decades younger than me, and he easily tipped the scales fifty pounds heavier—muscle, not fat. In the back of my mind, a whisper told me that age and size should mean nothing against technique. That whisper was drowned by the reality of inexperience, mine like a fledgling bird against his eagle's wings.

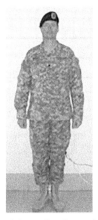

43-year-old me back in the Army
after being told I couldn't do that.

"Remember," the instructor barked, his voice slicing through the tense air, "this is about skill, not savagery. No blood, no broken teeth, and definitely no choking out."

We nodded, the ex-marine's eyes locked onto mine with military precision. There was something to learn here; to take a punch was to understand it, to dance with pain until it became just another step in the routine. This wasn't war, it was preparation for it, though every fiber in your body screamed otherwise when fists were flying.

As we circled each other, I thought about Shelly and Mandy waiting for me back home, their presence my anchor. If I could master these moves, endure this, then what couldn't I handle? The thought lent me strength, a hopeful note amid the symphony of aches that already played along my spine.

The ex-marine moved first, a feint that I narrowly countered. Our dance was one of near-misses and half-caught breaths, of exertion trembling on the edge of control. His blows were a thunderstorm I weathered, while mine felt like rain against a mountain. Yet there was a beauty in the struggle, a thread of resilience woven into the very fabric of our movements.

Every block, every strike taught me more about my limits—and how to push past them. The pain was a reminder, a sharp jab to my

147

consciousness that said I was still fighting, still standing, still moving forward.

"Good!" the instructor shouted from somewhere beyond the flurry of our exchange. "Keep it controlled, Quayle!"

And I did. With each passing second, luck seemed to weave itself into hope, threading through my veins with the promise that if I could just hold on, just keep going, then maybe I'd come out stronger on the other side.

Muscle against muscle, we grappled on the mat, each of us locked in a combat of strength and wits. I could feel his power, the sheer force of his youth pressing down on me, but there was something else at play within me—a quiet determination that age hadn't yet eroded. His height advantage meant nothing when I slipped behind him, hooking my arm around his neck in a rear-naked choke-hold. He struggled, a bear caught in a trap, but I had him. I didn't cinch the hold; I just needed him to know he was caught.

The others started jeering, their laughter a cruel symphony to this young giant's unexpected defeat. "C'mon, kid! Don't let Grandpa take you down!" they hollered. It was supposed to be a joke, light-hearted ribbing among soldiers, but as I held him there, immobilized yet unharmed, I saw it—the shift in his eyes. The humor of the moment drained away, leaving only that hollow, distant gaze. A thousand-yard stare that spoke of horrors seen and not forgotten.

"Easy," I murmured, more to myself than him, recognizing the signs of a wounded soul. My heart clenched with an unwelcome tightness, understanding that this was no longer about training or proving a point. It was about humanity. I released my grip and tapped out, signaling peace, retreat, end of the line.

But peace didn't come. Instead, he turned on me with a ferocity that belied his inner torment, pouncing like a cornered animal fighting for survival. Hands like vices, he came at me with a desperation born from a battlefield far from here, from a past that clung to him more tightly than any chokehold I could muster.

Three soldiers were pulling him back before I knew what happened, dragging him away as his punches fell like hailstones—unpredictable, relentless, uncontrollable. And amid that chaos, something gave way inside me. Not pride, not spirit, but something far more literal: my spine, in the area nearest my heart, yielding under a pressure it wasn't meant to withstand.

I lay there, breathing hard, the pain a growing chorus beneath my adrenaline-fueled shock. What had begun as a lesson had ended as a brutal reminder of the hidden battles we carry within us, the scars we don't always see.

Yet even as the realization of injury began to dawn, hope sprouted defiantly in its wake. This wasn't the end—not of me, not of this journey. Luck, that ever-present specter, hadn't abandoned me. It whispered in the recesses of my mind, promising that if I could rise above this, then nothing could ever truly hold me down.

"Quayle, you good?" someone asked, a distant voice through the ringing in my ears.

"Gettin' there," I replied, a statement more of intent than fact. Because giving up wasn't in my nature—not now, not ever. Even as I faced the unknown consequences of this day, I clung to the resilience that had brought me this far. Today's fall was merely the setup for tomorrow's rise. With every breath, hope grew stronger, and I knew that somehow, someway, I would stand again.

*****

The road to El Paso stretched out before us like a long, dusty promise. As Shelly guided her Prius ahead, Mandy's head occasionally popped up in the rearview mirror, as if checking on my progress. I followed in the U-Haul, its lumbering mass carrying not just our belongings but also the weight of my recent struggle. My back, a constant reminder of the incident at Fort Sill, protested with every jolt and bump of the truck. Yet there was solace in movement; it wasn't stillness but motion that kept the worst of the pain at bay.

I had been checked by the medics, their X-rays peering into me with cold precision and finding nothing amiss. "It's probably just a strain," they said, handing me a bottle of ibuprofen that might as well have been a placebo for all the good it did. "Report to duty tomorrow," they instructed, dismissing the pain that clung stubbornly to my spine. So I did what I had learned to do best over the years—I adapted, I adjusted, and I pressed on. I was no stranger to discomfort or to the relentless passage of time, having reached an age where youthful vigor was now a visitor rather than a resident within my body.

With each mile marker passed, my thoughts drifted to the resilience of those who had tread similar paths. The pioneers, the dreamers, the fighters—all those who had journeyed west with hopes as vast as the horizon. Here I was, following in their tireless footsteps, a modern man with an old warrior's heart.

Arriving in El Paso was like taking a deep breath after holding it for too long. The city welcomed us with open arms and a pressing heat that seemed to seep into every pore. I was grateful, though, for the chance to escape the confines of the driver's seat, to stand and stretch muscles that had cramped around an invisible vice. Movement was my ally, and I leaned into it, feeling the persistent ache in my back ease ever so slightly with each step I took.

In those moments, walking under the expansive Texas sky, I allowed myself to feel hopeful, hopeful that this new beginning in El Paso would be the salve I needed, not just for my physical wounds but for the deeper ones that couldn't be seen on any X-ray. Luck had carried me through thus far, a silent partner in my journey that nudged me forward when the odds seemed insurmountable.

Old-man-itis, I mused to myself, a wry smile tugging at the corner of my mouth. Age might slow me down, but it would never stop me. I could feel the chapters of my life turning, each page a testament to the trials faced and the victories hard-won. This pain, like every other obstacle before it, would not define me.

Instead, it would become another story I'd tell, another lesson I'd learn from. With each twinge in my back, I was reminded that life is not about avoiding the struggles but about facing them head-on, embracing them even. Because it's in the overcoming that we truly understand our strength. And as the sun dipped below the horizon, painting the desert in hues of fire and gold, I knew one thing for certain: I was not yet finished. There were still miles to go, still dreams to chase, and still a future to shape with these two resilient hands.

Stepping out of my SUV, I took a deep breath, the desert air dry and hot against my skin. The sun bore down on the base with an intensity that seemed to radiate off the tarmac in waves. For a moment, I stood still, letting my body acclimate to the sweltering heat of El Paso. With each pulse of pain from my back, I reminded myself, "This is just another test of your resolve, Bobby."

I reported for duty at the makeshift headquarters, a cluster of trailers huddled together like a caravan stranded in no man's land. The base was so new it felt like the ink had barely dried on the blueprints. As one of the first to don the insignia of this nascent brigade, I was stepping into a role that would demand every ounce of perseverance I had.

"Quayle," barked a voice from the trailer designated as our command post. "You're with the Cavalry Battalion, S-2 Shop."

The words were terse, the expectation clear. There was no time to wallow in discomfort; we had a brigade to build from the ground up.

The S-2 Shop was a hub of critical information, a place where the puzzle pieces of intelligence were assembled and presented to those who needed them most. Maintaining security clearances, analyzing threats, our purpose was vital, and I felt the weight of that responsibility settle on my shoulders. It was not just about holding the line; it was about foreseeing the dangers that lay beyond it.

The trailers were ovens, the metal walls trapping the heat inside until the very air you breathed felt thick and heavy. Sweat trickled down my spine, a relentless reminder of the environment's harshness. But within these confines, I found a sense of purpose that transcended physical discomfort. I poured over maps and reports, the ache in my back a mere footnote to the narrative of dedication unfolding within me.

Every day was a trial by fire, both literally and figuratively. Our equipment might have been sparse, our accommodations lacking, but what we lacked in resources we made up for in determination. We were pioneers in our own right, forging the path for those who would follow.

My hands, though calloused and worn, were tools of precision as I sifted through data, extracting the essential kernels of truth. My mind, trained to anticipate and strategize, adapted to the rhythm of military intelligence. In the quiet moments between briefings and debriefings, I could almost hear the history books being written, the pages filling with our efforts and triumphs.

In the vast expanse of the desert, under the unyielding gaze of the sun, I found an unexpected ally in hope. It was the kindle that sparked each morning when the fatigue clung to my limbs and the fuel that burned late into the night as I planned for the unknowns of tomorrow.

My journey was not just about overcoming physical adversity; it was about embracing the challenge before me with an unwavering spirit. I was shaping more than just a brigade; I was sculpting a legacy of resilience that would outlast even the strongest structures we were yet to build.

There, amid the dust and the relentless drone of activity, I forged a sense of camaraderie with my fellow soldiers—the shared understanding that what we were undertaking was greater than any one of us. This was where I belonged, where my story continued, and where my past tribulations became the foundation for future victories. And as the sun set each evening, casting its golden hue across the barren landscape, I could feel it deep in my bones: luck may have brought me here, but it was grit that would see me through.

The desert air was already simmering as I laced up my boots, the sun barely peeking over the horizon. It's funny how life can strip you down to your barest form, only to dress you in new armor. Here I was, Specialist E-4 once again, a humble rank that felt both like a demotion and a fresh start. But as the dust swirled around our makeshift operations center, I knew the stripes of a Sergeant E-5 weren't far out of reach. My hands, calloused and steady, were ready to earn back what time had taken.

"You should be a sergeant," said CPT Littles as he walked by, noticing the hard work that I was putting into the creation of this new brigade of ours.

"Thank you, sir!" I replied after saluting him. He was a good commander; he truly cared about his soldiers and always did his best to ensure that we were all well taken care of.

Every day was a marathon without a finish line in sight, a relentless push forward as we breathed life into this nascent brigade. The Army Corps of Engineers moved earth and stone with a symphony of machinery, crafting the skeleton of what would soon be a fully operational nerve center for warriors. Motor pools began to take shape, workshops rose from the ground, and barracks dotted the landscape like mirages promising respite.

In those eighteen months, sweat became as much a part of my uniform as the patches on my shoulder. I could feel the weight of responsibility on my back, heavier than any rucksack I'd carried before. Yet amid the clatter of construction and the grind of daily tasks, my resolve only hardened. This wasn't just about rebuilding; it was about proving—to myself and to the men and women at my side—that I still had the mettle to rise through the ranks.

Hope thrived here, a stubborn weed pushing through the cracks of parched soil. It wasn't just the anticipation of what this place would become but also the realization of what I was becoming alongside it. Each morning brought a renewed sense of purpose, each evening a reflection on the progress made, not just in erecting buildings but in fortifying the spirit of our unit.

There was a quiet pride in watching the physical transformation of the base, parallel to the inner growth I experienced. As I reclaimed the title of Sergeant, it was more than just the stripes on my sleeve— it was the reaffirmation that every setback was an opportunity in disguise, every challenge a chance to display the resilience etched deep within my core.

We built, we toiled, and we transformed—both the land and ourselves. With every sunrise that painted the sky with promise, I felt luck intertwine with determination, creating a tapestry of triumphs yet to come. And as the sun dipped below the rim of the world each night, I knew that tomorrow would be another step toward greatness, another chance to prove that hope is the most powerful tool in a soldier's arsenal.

The sun was just cresting over the Franklin Mountains when I stepped into the operations trailer, the hum of activity within a stark contrast to the silence of the dawn outside. After being promoted to Sergeant, I was given a new mission as the unit's Operations Sergeant or Training NCO, as some called it. In those early hours, the unit felt like a body waking up, each soldier a vital organ coming to life. My role was the nervous system, connecting every moving part, ensuring that the whole functioned seamlessly.

I pored over the training rosters with meticulous care, tracking the pulse of readiness that beat through our ranks. Weapons qualifications were up-to-date, physical fitness scores steadily improving, and mandatory training sessions checked off one by one. The rhythm of progress was palpable, a drumbeat that resonated with my own heart.

It was during this time, amid the strict regimen of military life, that I found an unexpected sanctuary at the El Paso Zoo. Volunteering there wasn't just about giving back; it became a balm for the soul, a place where simplicity met service, where nature's raw beauty could be touched, even if through bars.

There was one resident in particular who captured my affection, a gentle giant, an elephant named Maya. The first time her trunk enveloped me in an awkward yet tender embrace, I felt a connection that transcended species. It was as if she knew the weight on my shoulders and offered solace without judgment. Each time I fed her, swept her enclosure, or simply talked to her, the stress of my responsibilities seemed to dissipate, carried away on the desert breeze.

Then came the lion cubs, five bundles of energy and curiosity that arrived like a storm. The male, whom the staff had named Leo, was especially boisterous. Our games of tug of war became a highlight of my visits. His fierce little growls and determined tugs on the rope mirrored my own inner fight—playful yet a reminder of the wild strength within us all.

As I stood there in the zoo, matching pull for pull with Leo, I couldn't help but find parallels between these animals and my soldiers. Just like these cubs needed nurturing to grow strong, so did the men and women under my watch. And as Maya's trust had to be earned with patience and kindness, so did the respect of my team.

In those moments of laughter and shared determination, the hope that had carried me here blossomed. Luck might have played a hand in my journey, but it was resilience that shaped my path, hope that painted the horizon with endless possibilities. Standing there, the rope straining in my hands, I felt the unyielding promise of the future—a future I was helping to build, both within the confines of the base and the wider community beyond its gates.

The sun beat down on the back of my neck, a familiar sensation as I stood in formation. The heat was nothing new, but today it felt different—it was the warmth of recognition, not just from the blazing El Paso sun. My hands were steady at my sides, betraying none of the anticipation stirring within me.

"Today, we honor one of our own," Captain Littles's voice rang clear across the parade ground. As he pinned the Military Outstanding Volunteer Service Medal to my uniform, I could feel the weight of the small insignia, heavy with meaning, light in mass. It was a tangible testament to hours spent not in the line of fire, but in the service of compassion—feeding elephants, nurturing lion cubs, and witnessing the wide-eyed wonder of children as they came face-to-face with nature's marvels.

As Captain Littles pinned the medal on my chest, he said, "It seems that I have you up in front of the formation a lot lately. First the promotion, and now this award. Well done, Sergeant, keep up the great work!"

The applause of my comrades was a soothing balm, reaffirming that the work I'd done off base had rippled back to reflect positively on us all. This medal was more than a decoration; it was a bridge between the military community and the world beyond, built on mutual respect and understanding. Yet even as the metal gleamed on my chest, I knew it wasn't the accolade that filled me with pride—it was the joy I saw in those children's eyes when they beheld the animals. That was the reward no ceremony could match.

With the deployment looming, a different kind of resolve anchored itself in my heart. Approaching the first sergeant later that day, I shared my aspirations without hesitation. "I want to deploy as an intelligence analyst, not as an operations sergeant," I stated, my voice firm with conviction. My path to warrant officer school hinged on this deployment, and I believed my service warranted this opportunity.

"Your record speaks for itself," the first sergeant replied, his gaze reflecting the consideration I sought. Decorations aside, it was the silent battles, the relentless grind, and the unyielding hope that truly defined my tenure here.

As I walked away, the future stretched out before me—a tableau of challenges and chances. It was a future I would meet head-on with the resilience that had carried me through pain and uncertainty and the hope that whispered promises of triumph yet to come. In my mind's eye, I saw Leo, the lion cub now grown, his playful tugs transformed into the majestic strength of a fully-fledged roar. Like him, I would stand tall, ready to embrace whatever lay ahead.

And as the sun dipped below the horizon, casting long shadows over the base, I couldn't help but smile, buoyed by the prospect of what tomorrow might bring. Luck had brought me here, but it would be grit and determination that would see me through.

The weight on my back was as familiar as the ache that threaded through my spine. With each step, I could feel the gravel crunch beneath my boots while the rucksack seemed to press its heavy contents into my muscles like an unyielding reminder of what I had signed up for. The desert sun beat down mercilessly. The heat was a tangible force, but it was not enough to burn away the determination that simmered within me.

"Keep moving, Bobby," I muttered to myself, the words a silent mantra that matched the rhythm of my march. These long ruck marches were my battleground, and every mile conquered was a victory against the insidious voice that whispered doubts fueled by my persistent back pain. It was during these moments of solitary struggle when I felt closest to Sergeant Martinez's example of unwavering resilience. Her strength, though she wasn't here, spurred me on.

When the news came down from my commander and first sergeant—that my request to deploy as an intelligence analyst hung in limbo—I knew this was yet another obstacle to overcome, not a defeat. "It's out of our hands," they had said with sympathetic shrugs. But sympathy wouldn't guide my career; action would.

Taking their advice, I invoked the open-door policy, standing before the brigade sergeant major with the same resolve that carried me through the marches. The clink of my medals, including the one awarded for my volunteer work at the zoo, was a soft chorus underpinning my quiet confidence. I laid out my case with the clarity of someone who understood the stakes—not just for myself but for the unit.

"Understood, Sergeant," the sergeant major had finally said, his nod slow, contemplative. "You'll transfer to the intelligence battalion and deploy with them."

As I left his office, the sense of hope that bloomed within me was as real and vibrant as the El Paso sunsets that painted the sky with strokes of fiery passion. I had faced many trials, the physical toll on my body being just one. Yet it was the hopeful persistence, the belief in the value of my dreams, that lifted me above the ache in my back and propelled me forward.

I thought about the future, picturing myself in the field, gathering intelligence, making decisions that could save lives. It was more than a role; it was a calling, one that demanded my all.

With only a week left before the transfer, my mind was alight with preparations, but my heart paused to reflect on the journey. There was no room for "old-man-itis," not when purpose coursed through my veins. This was my fight, my mission. And as I shouldered my rucksack once more, the weight felt less like a burden and more like the armor of a warrior ready for the fray.

The morning dawned just like any other in the relentless heat of El Paso, but this day held a different kind of promise. A week away from my transfer to the Intelligence Battalion—a move that would shape my future career—I was determined to meet every challenge head-on. Today's challenge wasn't a strategic puzzle or a clandestine report, it was something far more visceral: a three-mile run with my soldier, PFC Murphy, and the first sergeant.

"Keep up if you can," the first sergeant had thrown down the gauntlet with a wry grin as he stretched his muscular arms across his chest. He was a formidable runner, his reputation well known among the ranks. But today, there was a flicker of something else in my chest—pride, perhaps, or maybe the stubborn streak that had carried me through countless hurdles.

"You might be the one lagging behind, Top," I retorted, trying to sound more confident than I felt.

My back, a constant reminder of a past hidden beneath layers of uniform and stoic resolve, screamed its protest. I breathed through the pain, focusing on the task at hand. As we set off, I could almost feel the fibers in my muscles warming, loosening, the ache in my spine dulling with each determined stride. My soldier fell into pace beside me, and together, we found our rhythm, our footsteps a drumbeat on the pavement.

The first sergeant was right there with us, a silent shadow pushing us to go faster, be better. In those moments, the run became more than physical training; it was a testament to willpower, to refusing to be outpaced by life's relentless march. With the wind slicing past, creating a symphony with the thudding of my heartbeat, I let the world blur into a backdrop for my focus.

Then, without warning, a curious sensation shivered through me. It began as a tingling at the base of my neck, like the whisper of an unforeseen change in the weather. Down my spine it danced, a peculiar, electrifying feeling that seemed to carry both foreboding and relief in its wake. As it reached my legs, the sensation morphed, growing stranger still, as if my limbs were suddenly speaking a language my mind couldn't quite comprehend.

I pressed on, chasing the fleeting comfort that running had brought me moments before. The first sergeant's steady breaths were close, a metronome to my own increasingly erratic ones. This was a new kind of pain, not the familiar companion I had begrudgingly accepted, but an intruder with mysterious intentions.

As I ran, hope twined with uncertainty. The path ahead was as unknown as the sensations now racing through my body, yet I clung to the resilience that had carried me here, to this place, to this moment. For even as challenges loomed, I knew that hope was the torch that illuminated the darkest roads, the beacon that guided wearied travelers home.

I thought of Sergeant Martinez, her quick wit and steadfast courage, how her loyalty never faltered when faced with adversity. She'd often say, "Adversity introduces us to ourselves," and in that instant, I understood her words with crystalline clarity. I was more than my rank, more than my pain—I was a soldier, unyielding and resolute.

With every step, I reaffirmed my commitment to the journey, no matter how treacherous the terrain. This ache was just another adversary, one I would confront with the same tenacity that had become my signature. I was a man who thrived against the odds, who saw the finish line not as the end but as the starting point of the next great race.

And so I ran—not away from the pain or toward an uncertain future but alongside the ever-present hope that propelled me through life's marathon, where every heartache was a hurdle cleared and every victory was a testament to the indomitable human spirit.

The gravel crunched under my uncooperative feet, each step growing heavier than the last. A dull ache radiated from my back, a mocking reminder of the youthful vigor I once possessed and the relentless march of time. Sweat beaded on my brow, not just from exertion but also from a creeping dread as my legs began to betray me.

"Are you okay, Sarge?" Private Murphy's voice cut through the haze of my focus.

My legs, they weren't just heavy; they were rebelling, refusing the commands issued by a brain that could not fathom this sudden mutiny. "Your legs, they are moving funny, what's wrong?" Murphy's query echoed again, concern lacing his tone, pulling me into the sharp light of reality. The truth was I didn't know—couldn't understand—why my body was faltering beneath me.

"Murphy," I grunted, pride wrestling with the fear that threatened to swallow me whole, "just...stay close."

"I can carry you back if you need me to, Sarge," he offered, the loyalty in his eyes shining brighter than the morning sun glinting off the distant barracks, but I had a feeling that being slung over his shoulders was a very bad idea.

I shook my head, a soldier's stubbornness surging within me. "No, just be ready. I may need your shoulder."

We trudged on, my once-firm strides reduced to an awkward shuffle, Private Murphy a steadfast shadow at my side. Time stretched, warping around us until the offices appeared like a mirage on the horizon, our sanctuary from the unforgiving terrain.

As we approached, the first sergeant's figure loomed, returning from the run, his presence commanding even in stillness. His eyes, sharp as ever, immediately registered the situation. "What's going on, Sergeant?" The worry in his voice was unfamiliar yet comforting, like a rare desert bloom.

"Legs aren't…cooperating," I managed, my energy waning but not my resolve. There was no room for surrender, not now, not ever. This was but another obstacle, a testament to endurance, to the resilience that had become part of my very essence.

And though fear gnawed at the edges of my mind, hope remained steadfast in its vigil. For I was reminded of the words of Sergeant Martinez, her strength woven into the fabric of my being: "Adversity introduces us to ourselves." These legs, this pain, it was merely an introduction to another facet of my spirit—a spirit unyielding.

With every labored breath, I clung to the belief that this was just another chapter in my story, a narrative punctuated by trials but defined by triumphs. And as the first sergeant's strong hand grasped my arm, steadying me, I knew that whatever lay ahead, I would face it with the same indomitable will that had carried me thus far.

For I am a soldier—not of rank or title but of heart and soul—and no injury, no setback, could dim the bright flame of hope that fueled my every step forward.

*****

The sterile scent of the hospital mingled with the low hum of machinery as I lay there, trying to make sense of the persistent numbness in my legs. The gentle click of the door announced the arrival of the medical team, their faces etched with a professional concern that did little to ease the knot of anxiety in my stomach.

"Did you know that your spine is fractured?" one of the doctors asked, pulling up images that seemed to belong to someone else's life, not mine. The screen flickered to life, revealing the ghostly outline of my own backbone—a jagged line where smooth continuity should have been. "It's right here at T-7 and T-8, near your heart," a doctor explained, her finger hesitating over the aberration that had stealthily undermined my strength.

Confusion reigned as I cast my mind back, searching for the moment of impact that could explain such an injury. No car crashes or falls came to mind, only the ever-present ache that had become as familiar as my own shadow. Then, like a lightning strike, realization dawned—the combat training, the grapple with the ex-marine whose eyes held wars I could never fathom.

"Wait a minute!" The words tumbled from my lips before I could corral them, the pieces falling into place with a clarity that was both liberating and chilling. Over eighteen long months, my body had borne the silent testimony of that day, carrying the burden of an invisible wound while I pushed it to its limits, preparing for a deployment to Afghanistan that now seemed as distant as the stars above.

"Do you have any idea how lucky you are, Sergeant?" The question hung in the air, a testament to what could have been lost. The doctor's gaze met mine, filled with a mixture of astonishment and respect. It was a sobering thought—how close I had come to a fate that would have left me a mere observer in my own life.

Mr. Magoo strikes again, I thought as the doctor explained the extent of the injury.

Yet even as the gravity of the situation settled upon my shoulders like winter's first snow, hope kindled within me, refusing to be extinguished. For luck had been my shadow, too, guiding me through the unknowable maze of close calls and happenstance that had delivered me to this point. Each step I had taken was a dance with chance, leading me to a precipice from which I could now see the true measure of my resilience.

In the quiet of that room, with the soft beeps and whirs of machines charting the path of my heartbeat, I found solace in the knowledge that every challenge surmounted had fortified my spirit, preparing me for this new battle. There would be no white flags, no conceding despair; only the steadfast belief that, against all odds, I would rise again.

For in the crucible of adversity, hope is the strongest metal, and I was forged from nothing less. My story was not one of unbroken triumphs but of perseverance, of finding light in the darkest of times. And as I lay there, contemplating the road ahead, I knew that whatever may come, I would face it head-on, bolstered by the unwavering conviction that only through embracing our struggles do we truly learn what it means to prevail.

The cool, antiseptic scent of the hospital room pressed against my senses as I grappled with the surgeon's words. The chill that crept into my bones wasn't from the sterile air—it was fear, raw and biting. But beneath that ice, a fire was kindling, a fierce defiance that refused to be smothered.

"You will need surgery, and there is a chance that you may not be able to walk again," he explained with clinical detachment. The words ricocheted inside my skull, an echo chamber of potential loss.

"Fuck you, sir," I spat, the pain medication loosening my tongue and inflaming my temper. "I'm walking out of this hospital! With all due respect, sir, I WILL walk again!" My voice was a growl, a primal claim over my own fate.

The doctor, taken aback but composed, understood the tumult within me. "I hope you do walk out of here, Sergeant," he said, signaling for the nurses. "Prepare him for surgery."

*****

Those seventy-five days following were a blur of agony and determination. Each morning brought new challenges, each evening small victories. The rehabilitation center became my battleground, the therapists my comrades-in-arms, guiding me through the relentless drills that would reforge the connection between mind and muscle.

"Push through it, Bobby," they'd say, their voices firm yet encouraging. And I did. I pushed through the sweat and the tears, through the moments when my legs trembled like saplings in a storm, refusing to hold my weight. I willed them to obey, to remember their strength.

"It's not about how hard you can hit, it's about how hard you can get hit and keep moving forward. That's how winning is done!" Rocky Balboa's gritty mantra pounded in my head with every faltering step I took on the treadmill. Those simple words became my anthem, urging me onward.

There were days when the light seemed to flicker and dim, when the shadows of doubt whispered of surrender. But then I'd recall the faces of the soldiers I'd served with—and I knew I couldn't give up. They had fought their battles, and now, so must I.

As I lay in bed at night, my body aching from the day's exertions, I'd think about my journey: the relentless back pain, the unexpected diagnosis, the sudden pivot my life had taken. It struck me then, the sheer randomness of life, the way luck dances with us all—sometimes leading, sometimes following.

I clung to hope like a shield, letting it armor me against despair. I filled my thoughts with visions of walking Mandy in the park, of stepping alongside Shelly, each stride a testament to perseverance. Through that lens of hope, I saw not a world defined by limitations but one rich with possibility.

When the day came to leave the hospital, my departure was not marked by fanfare or ceremony. There was only the quiet triumph of placing one foot in front of the other, each step a declaration. As the automatic doors slid open, a breeze kissed my face, whispering of newfound horizons waiting just beyond the threshold.

I stepped into the sunlight, squinting against its brilliance, a free man once more. The road ahead was uncertain, sure to be lined with obstacles and trials. Yet I felt a surge of elation, for I knew whatever came, I would meet it head-on. I had been tested, shaped by adversity, and emerged with a deeper understanding of my own strength.

And so I walked on, each step a pulse in the rhythm of my recovery, a beat in the heart of a story still unfolding—a tale of resilience, of luck's fickle hand, and of hope's undying light.

The sun was already high in the sky, casting a warm glow over the base as I limped across the parking lot to begin the transition out of the life I had known. The weight of my medical files in my backpack felt like an anchor, each page a reminder of the dreams that now seemed so distant. Yet in every step, there was a quiet defiance—a refusal to be defined by the injuries that threatened to claim my military career.

As I entered the administrative building for my initial meeting, the sterile scent of polished floors and the sound of hushed voices created a stark contrast to the chaos of the battlefield. I thought back to the days when I donned my uniform with pride, when the rhythm of cadence calls matched the beat of my heart. But those days were gone, and in their place was a future unwritten, a blank slate upon which I would have to inscribe a new purpose.

Sitting down across from the medical board officer, a man with sharp eyes and a meticulously organized desk, I could sense the gravity of what was about to unfold. His voice was even and practiced as he began explaining the medical evaluation and retirement process. It was a labyrinth of paperwork, evaluations, and waiting—so much waiting. There was no combat strategy that could prepare me for this battle, one fought with pens and patience rather than prowess and physicality.

"Mr. Quayle," he said, breaking into my thoughts, "I understand this is not how you envisioned ending your service." His words were meant to comfort, but they hung in the air like a question I wasn't ready to answer. I nodded, my throat tight, acknowledging the truth in his statement.

I left the office with a stack of documents and a heavy heart. The path ahead was fraught with unknowns, and yet within me stirred a determination that had been forged in the crucible of adversity. The same resolve that had carried me through the grueling hours of therapy propelled me now, reminding me that while my role in the army was concluding, my journey was far from over.

It would be easy to succumb to bitterness, to let the what-ifs consume me, but I chose instead to look forward, to see each challenge as a steppingstone rather than a stumbling block. I envisioned myself not as a soldier sidelined by injury but as a warrior of the spirit, battling for a different kind of victory—one measured in small triumphs and personal growth.

In the evenings, as I sat on the porch with Shelly, watching the hues of dusk paint the sky, I shared my fears and my hopes. Her hand in mine was a lifeline, her belief in me a beacon guiding me through the uncertainty. Together, we planned and dreamed, crafting a vision of a future where my experiences in the army were not an end but a foundation upon which we could build something new, something meaningful.

"Whatever happens, we'll face it together," Shelly said, her voice steady and sure. In that moment, I felt luck's gentle nudge, a whisper of fate that reminded me that no matter the hardship, I was never alone. With each sunrise and sunset, I found solace in the consistency of nature's cycles, the promise that after every night comes the dawn.

And so as I faced the arduous process of medical retirement, I did so with an introspective eye and a hopeful heart. My story was not one of a fall from grace but of transformation, a tale of a man who, when confronted with the specter of defeat, chose instead to rise, time and again, fueled by resilience, hope, and the steadfast belief in second chances.

CHAPTER 14

A PAINFUL INJURY

I remember walking into the sterile, nondescript room of the Intelligence Battalion for the first time since my transfer—every step a silent testament to the pain and determination that had brought me back on my feet. The surgery scars were hidden beneath my uniform, but the apprehension was etched plainly across my face. My identity within these walls was as new and fragile as the healing bones in my back; I was an unknown entity, a puzzle yet to be placed within their ranks.

The air was thick with the skepticism that comes easily to those trained to question everything. I could feel the weight of their stares, the unvoiced questions that hung between us like a fog. They didn't know about the countless hours I'd spent in rehabilitation, relearning the rhythm of putting one foot in front of the other. They didn't see the resolve that had driven me to meet personally with the brigade sergeant major, advocating for myself to secure this transfer. My dream had been clear: to serve in Afghanistan as an intelligence analyst, not behind a desk as an operations sergeant. My ambition had been fueled by a desire to engage more directly with the mission, to contribute in a manner that resonated with my own calling.

But dreams have a way of unraveling when faced with reality. When the news broke that I wouldn't be deploying with the unit, a murmur of betrayal snaked its way through the barracks. It was a crushing blow; the very foundation of my transfer had crumbled beneath me. Whispers swelled into hostile glares, each one a dagger suggesting that maybe, just maybe, I had orchestrated this outcome to avoid the perils of deployment.

"Nichols," I called out softly, my voice barely above the hum of the busy operations center.

Sergeant Nichols glanced up from her workstation, her sharp eyes quickly taking in my troubled expression. She offered a subtle nod, an acknowledgment that she too had noticed the shift in demeanor around us. "Rough day?" she asked, her tone low, meant only for my ears.

"Seems like it's open season on assumptions," I replied, forcing a wry smile.

"Let them talk," Nichols said, her voice firm with the conviction I desperately needed. "We know the truth."

Her words were a lifeline thrown across the chasm of doubt that threatened to swallow me whole. In that moment, I clung fiercely to the hope that eventually, my intentions would shine brighter than the suspicions cast upon me. I had to believe that resilience, not resignation, would define my story.

As I made my way back to my workspace, the echo of my footsteps mingled with the relentless drumbeat of my heart. Each beat was a reminder that I was still here, still fighting, still hopeful. The road ahead might be marred by adversity, but I was no stranger to overcoming the insurmountable.

And so with every ounce of courage I could muster, I resolved to prove them wrong—not through words but through the unwavering dedication to my duty. Despite the hostility, despite the disappointment, I would not be deterred. For in the crucible of challenge, I knew, lay the opportunity to forge an indomitable spirit.

The weight of their glares was almost tangible as I entered the room, a thick fog of judgment that seemed to press against my every step. It was as if I had become a specter in my own life, haunting the corridors of a place I once called home within the military. The murmurs fell into an oppressive silence, and I knew what thoughts were marching through their minds: there goes the man who couldn't hack it, the soldier feigning injury to avoid the fight.

I used to wear my uniform with pride, the medals on my chest a testament to years of service and sacrifice. Now each ribbon felt like a shard of glass, a reminder of honor now questioned, of valor doubted by those who never saw the battles I faced or the scars they left behind.

"Quayle," the voice cut through the quiet, sharp and devoid of warmth. I turned to face the speaker, Sergeant Major Clarke, his eyes scrutinizing me as if searching for some crack in my resolve, any excuse to validate their misconceptions. "Make sure those reports are on my desk by 1600."

"Understood, Sergeant Major," I responded, my voice steady despite the turmoil churning within. I had learned to steel myself against the onslaught of skepticism, to shore up the defenses around my battered morale. But even the strongest walls have their limits, and I could feel the fissures growing with each passing day.

Walking past the rows of desks, I caught snippets of conversations abruptly hushed, sidelong glances quickly averted. The culture of suspicion had infiltrated every corner of this battalion, turning comrades into judges, brothers-in-arms into inquisitors. My injury, invisible to the naked eye but agonizingly present, was a mark of shame in their eyes. To them, I was just another malingerer, though nothing could be further from the truth.

Sitting down at my workstation, I let out a breath I hadn't realized I'd been holding. I thought back to the days when I was lauded as a hero, when my contributions were celebrated rather than questioned. Those memories now seemed like relics from another era, artifacts of a time when my worth wasn't measured by my ability to stand at attention or march into battle.

But self-pity was a luxury I couldn't afford. If there was one thing my journey had taught me, it was the power of resilience—the unyielding force of a spirit unwilling to break. They could cast their stones, erect their barriers, but they could not erode the foundation of determination upon which I built my life.

My fingers danced across the keyboard, compiling the intelligence reports that would still bear my name and my dedication to duty. I worked with meticulous care, knowing that in the end, my work would speak louder than their whispers. My commitment, undiminished by their disdain, would stand as a testament to my enduring loyalty to the mission, to the country I served.

And so I pressed on, buoyed by an inner hope that refused to be extinguished. Each keystroke was a defiant drumbeat, an affirmation that I was more than their doubts, greater than their scorn. In the crucible of their hostility, I found a renewed purpose—a chance to prove that courage comes not only from the battlefield but also from the quiet resolve to face adversity head-on, without flinching, without faltering.

"Quayle," Nichols's voice broke through my concentration. "You're doing good work here."

"Thanks, Nichols," I replied, grateful for the solidarity in her words. She understood the value of endurance, the strength born of facing down demons both external and internal.

With each day's close, I held fast to the belief that this chapter of my life, no matter how dark, would lead to a dawn of new beginnings. Beyond the confines of this office, beyond the narrow views of those who doubted me, lay possibilities as boundless as the sky. And it was to that horizon I set my sights, unwavering in my journey toward redemption and renewal.

As the first light of dawn crept through the slats of my bedroom blinds, I felt the weight of scrutiny bearing down on me. Every morning was like stepping onto a stage where every act and gesture was subject to interpretation by an audience eager for a slip-up. While comrades in arms should have stood shoulder to shoulder, there I was, isolated beneath a spotlight of suspicion.

I laced up my boots with methodical precision, each loop and knot a small battle won against the day's looming challenges. My body ached from the past—remnants of surgery and the relentless grind of recovery—but it also bore the scars of judgment, heavier and more cumbersome than any physical injury.

"Keep your head high, Quayle," I murmured to myself, a mantra for the moments when doubt crept in like an unwelcome shadow. The mirror reflected someone who had been chiseled by adversity, a man whose uniform hung differently now, strained across a frame that had borne the brunt of life's crueler twists.

The walk to the office was a gauntlet. Eyes followed me, whispers fluttering behind closed doors like moths to a flame. Yet it was not weakness they saw—it was resilience. Each step was a testament to my commitment, a silent rebuttal to those who watched, hoping for a falter.

At my desk, the paperwork stacked high—a tangible measure of time and persistence. They had tried to add the burden of numbers to my file, a misguided attempt to use my weight as a weapon against me. But regulations are clear-cut defenses, shields against the onslaught of bias and unfounded accusations. My pending retirement was a fortress wall that no misguided attempt could breach.

"Dismiss their ignorance," I coached myself, fingers flying over the keyboard as I compiled reports, analysis that still mattered, work that still contributed to something greater than myself. It was my contribution that defined me, not the capricious opinions of those who could not fathom the depth of my dedication.

In the quiet hum of computers and the distant sounds of orders being given, I found a strange solace. This was not just about enduring; it was about prevailing. Despite the long shadow cast by misunderstanding, hope glimmered—a beacon that promised a future unshackled from the present's turmoil.

Each document sealed and sent was another step forward, a quiet victory in a war waged within the confines of bureaucracy. The resilience that had seen me through combat now fortified me in this new theater, one where the enemy wore the same uniform but lacked the same honor.

"Quayle," came the occasional acknowledgments from those few who understood the struggle, their voices like lifelines cast across choppy waters. Replies were sparse, nods of gratitude for the recognition of worth still intact.

And so I held steadfast to a vision of tomorrow, one shaped by the hope of what lay beyond this chapter. In the vast expanse of what was yet to come, I saw a life reclaimed, a narrative rewritten not by the hands of others but by my own determination and the unwavering support of those who truly knew me.

A new day beckoned on the horizon, one where the shadows of the past would be outshone by the light of a new purpose. With each tick of the clock, I edged closer to that dawn, to the promise of peace earned not only through service but also through the strength to stand tall amid the storm.

The chill of the early morning air had become a familiar sensation as I made my way to the Brigade Operations Center, the sky just beginning to lighten with the promise of a new day. It was 7:45 when I entered the building, the quiet hum of the operations room greeting me like an old friend. In fifteen minutes exactly, I would stand before the Brigade Commander, delivering the intelligence report with precision, despite the storm that raged within the unit I represented.

My mind, always racing ahead, couldn't help but fixate on the absurdity of the situation. The first sergeant, dogged in his determination to see me ousted, had scheduled the unit weigh-in for the exact time of my briefing. There was a certain perverse irony in the fact that my commitment to duty, reporting to the commander at eight o'clock sharp, was being used against me. But the regulations were clear; I was exempt due to my medical retirement process. Yet regulations seemed to matter little in this personal vendetta cloaked in military discipline.

As I concluded my briefing and watched the commander nod appreciatively, I felt a small surge of validation. Walking out at 8:25, I steeled myself for the next confrontation. As expected, upon arrival at the intelligence unit, the atmosphere was charged with silent accusations. I ignored the murmurs, making my way to the scales for the post-briefing weigh-in, adhering to orders, even as they were weaponized against me.

"Nichols," I called softly, seeking the eyes of the one ally among the sea of skeptics. Sergeant Nichols offered a slight nod, her presence a subtle yet potent reminder that not all judged so harshly. We shared no words; none were needed. Her understanding fortified me, a testament to the unspoken bond between those who have weathered similar trials.

The resilience borne of years in service, of challenges faced and overcome, now wove itself into the fabric of my present circumstance. I knew the measure of my worth was not found in the numbers displayed on that scale nor in the skewed perceptions of those who sought my downfall. Hope flickered, undiminished by the shadows cast by doubt and malice, fueled by the knowledge that every end is simply the precursor to a new beginning.

With each step taken toward what lay ahead, I embraced the notion that adversity was but a crucible, shaping strength from the raw ore of experience. I carried within me not only the weight of my past but also the lightness of potential, of dreams yet realized. And as the sun crested the horizon, its rays scattering the remnants of darkness, I too looked toward the horizon, where my future awaited, unfettered by the chains of the present turmoil.

The crisp morning air bit at my cheeks as I walked toward the Brigade Operations Center, my mind a carousel of duty rosters and intelligence briefs. The sky above mirrored the turmoil within me, shades of gray wrestling with the promise of sunlight, hinting at clarity yet to break through.

"Morning, Sarge," I greeted the guard with a practiced smile, my voice steady despite the tempest brewing in my core.

"Good morning," he returned, his eyes carrying the weight of understanding. He knew of my struggle, a testament to the silent whispers that darted like shadows through the ranks. I entered the command center, saluting the American flag that stood proudly in the corner, its stars and stripes a reminder of the ideals I had pledged to uphold. I approached the brigade commander's desk, reports in hand, ready to fulfill my duties. But today was different; today was the day the first sergeant's persistence would unravel before the highest authority in our unit.

"Let's see the report," the brigade commander beckoned, his presence commanding yet not unkind. As I relayed the latest intelligence, a commotion stirred at the entrance. The first sergeant stormed in, brandishing what appeared to be my latest counseling statement, his face flushed with indignation. Undeterred by protocol, he thrust the document toward the commander as if it were Excalibur itself, capable of cutting down any who opposed him.

"Sir, this soldier has repeatedly failed to—" he began, but the commander cut him off with a gesture both swift and final.

"First Sergeant," he said, his voice resonating with authority, "my office, now."

Confusion etched into the first sergeant's features as the commander took the paper, examining it briefly before tearing it into pieces, the sound echoing through the room like a clap of thunder. My heart raced, each tear a release from the chains of baseless accusations and relentless scrutiny.

"Now," the commander spoke again, directing the first sergeant toward the door with a nod that brooked no argument. The door closed behind them with a click, sealing the fate of the man who had sought my demise with such fervor. It was public, it was decisive, and it reverberated through the walls of the very institution that had become my battlefield.

Later, I learned of his transfer, a whisper of justice in an otherwise deafening silence. Yet even as that chapter closed, the damage inscribed upon my spirit could not simply be erased. The weeks of surveillance, the underlying tension, the expectation of betrayal—it had manifested itself in more than just physical pain. A diagnosis now accompanied my name: acute anxiety and major depressive disorder. Labels that, while validating my unseen wounds, also deepened the scars.

Sitting in the small examination room, the white walls closing in, I clutched the medical report as though it were a lifeline. This piece of paper acknowledged the invisible enemy that had been tightening its grip around me. It was proof that the battle wounds were not solely the ones that marred flesh and bone.

As I stepped back into the daylight, the sun finally breaking through the clouds, I allowed myself a moment of respite. Despite everything, my spirit endured, a resilient flame flickering defiantly against the storm. There was hope yet a path forward beyond the field of conflict. "Tomorrow is another day," I whispered to myself, a mantra to soothe the restless echoes of my mind. The journey ahead might be fraught with uncertainty, but I was no stranger to adversity. And as I watched the sunrise paint the sky with hues of gold and amber, I believed, perhaps for the first time in a long while, that there was light after darkness, healing after hurt, life after service.

Leaning against the cool metal of my locker, I let out a sigh that seemed to carry the weight of the world. The whispers had become roars in the confines of the barracks, echoes of judgment that knew nothing of the truth. They didn't see the countless nights spent staring at the ceiling, willing my body to heal, to be fit for the mission I had trained for, the deployment I had sought with every fiber of my being.

"Quayle," a voice cut through the clamor, snapping me back to the present. Sergeant Nichols stood there, her expression tight with concern. "Ignore them," she said, though her eyes betrayed the futility of such advice.

"I never wanted this," I confided, the frustration boiling over as I turned to face her. "I didn't choose to be injured. All I wanted was to serve alongside my unit in Afghanistan."

She nodded, her hand finding its way to my shoulder in a rare gesture of solidarity. "I know you did, Bobby. And so do a few others who still remember what you're made of." But her words were a drop in an ocean of doubt, and I found myself floundering amid the waves of disdain from those who should have been my comrades-in-arms. There was a cruel irony to it all, a soldier once commended for his strength now perceived as feigning weakness. I shook my head, trying to dispel the rumors that clung to me like a second skin.

"It's not as if you can fake a fractured spine," I muttered more to myself than to anyone else.

The corridors of the base, once a symbol of unity and purpose, now felt like a labyrinth designed to trap me in a cycle of despair. Disgust curled within me, a visceral reaction to the juvenile culture that fostered such venom toward those down on their luck. The illness and injuries that befell soldiers were not choices, yet here we were, treated as pariahs for the sin of being human. My gaze fell upon the commendations that lined the insides of my locker door, mementos of a time when my worth was measured by my ability to stand firm in the face of adversity. That resilience had not waned, but the battlefield had shifted from the tangible to the intangible. Now the enemy was the very institution I had pledged my life to protect. "Retirement can't come soon enough," I whispered, almost as a prayer.

There was a life waiting for me beyond these gates, a chance to rebuild and restore what had been lost in the line of duty. It was a hope that glimmered faintly on the horizon, a guiding star in the darkest night. As I closed the locker, its solid clang serving as punctuation to my resolve, I allowed a moment of reflection.

My journey had been fraught with storms, but each tempest had taught me the value of pressing forward, of finding the eye where calm prevailed. And though the winds of change howled with uncertainty, I was ready to set sail toward new beginnings, leaving behind the shadows cast by old uniforms and outdated prejudices. With each step toward the exit, my heart grew lighter, the burden of unwarranted shame slipping from my shoulders. There would be no looking back, only the steadfast march toward a future where my narrative was my own to pen, where the chapters of my life were defined not by injury but by the indomitable spirit that had carried me through so much.

"Goodbye," I murmured to the empty hallway, my voice a harbinger of the dawn awaiting me. As I passed through the threshold, the sun's rays kissed my cheeks, a warm embrace bidding me farewell from a chapter that had closed and welcoming me to the blank pages yet to be written. I turned the letter over in my hands, its weight far heavier than the paper it was printed on. The embossed seal of commendation felt like a cruel joke—a reminder of what could have been but was now lessened, tarnished by disdain and bureaucratic spite. A lesser medal for over fifteen years of service—it was both an insult and a testament to the struggles I had faced. But within me, a fire of determination smoldered. This wasn't the end.

"Can you believe this, Shelly?" I asked, forcing a chuckle that didn't quite mask the sting. "After all these years, they downgraded the medal."

She looked at me, her eyes soft with understanding. "It's just not fair," she whispered, reaching across the table to squeeze my hand. "But you know your worth, Bobby. And so do I." Her support was a balm to the raw edges of my spirit. It was true; the medal didn't define me. My worth wasn't tied to the fabric of a uniform or the medal pinned upon my chest. I was more than that. I was a survivor, a warrior who had weathered storms and emerged, though battered, still standing.

The grueling, two-and-a-half-year-long process was finally coming to an end. After countless medical exams that involved a lot of poking and prodding, covering every aspect of my physical and mental health, the results were concerning. The doctor sat across from me in his office for the final exam before discharge, explaining the news. "We found twenty-seven different issues that you are rated disabled for by military standards," he stated grimly.

My heart sank as I listened to the list of disabilities. Spinal fracture at 50 percent, sleep apnea at 50 percent, hearing loss and tinnitus at 10 percent, depression and anxiety at a staggering 70 percent. The words washed over me, each one carrying its own weight of struggle and pain.

That night, as I sat down with Shelly to explain the doctors' notes and ratings, I could feel the weight of it all pressing down on me. But then, like a ray of sunshine breaking through the clouds, I remembered something else I wanted to tell her. "Hey, listen," I said, shifting the topic to brighter shores, "I found something—a chance for us to start anew." A spark of hope ignited within me as I spoke, a spring of possibility breaking through the hardened soil of adversity. "There are these franchises that are veteran-friendly, and there's an opportunity back in Ohio." A glimmer of excitement danced in my eyes as I shared this new prospect with her, determined to find a way forward despite the challenges we faced.

"Really?" Her eyes lit up, mirroring the spark of my own enthusiasm. "That sounds promising."

"Yeah," I nodded, feeling the weight of the past begin to lift. "And it's close to our families too. We could put down roots, build something of our own."

"I like that," she said, her smile growing. "And I've been thinking… Maybe I can go back to social work. Help people again, you know?"

"Helping others while building our future," I mused aloud, the concept taking shape, forming a vision of a life where purpose and passion could coexist. "It's perfect, Shelly."

We talked long into the night, spinning dreams from the threads of hardship and resilience. Our words wove a tapestry of a tomorrow filled with promise, a world where the shadows of yesterday no longer held sway.

The road ahead would be paved with challenges; I had no illusions about that. But with Shelly by my side, and the lessons etched into my soul by time and trial, I felt a burgeoning sense of confidence. I was ready to face the uncertainty, to embrace the fortunes that lay hidden just beyond the bend.

"Here's to new beginnings," I said, raising my glass in a silent toast to the horizon that awaited us.

"New beginnings," Shelly echoed, her voice rich with the music of hope.

As we settled into the comforting rhythm of shared plans, I knew that this was the turning point, the moment where the page would turn and a new chapter would begin. For every soldier knows that the true battle is not in the fighting but in the enduring. And endure we would, into a future bright with the light of untold dawns.

The California sun glinted off the polished sign that heralded my arrival at the franchise headquarters. It was a beacon, drawing me toward a future I had fought to claim—a symbol of the victories small and large that one accumulates like medals in the theater of life's battles. The air was thick with the scent of opportunity, and with each step I took toward the entrance, I could feel the weight of my past service lighten upon my shoulders.

Inside, the walls were adorned with photographs of other franchisees, their smiles broad beneath eyes alight with the same spark I felt igniting within me. The training room buzzed with the low hum of conversation, a collective murmur of aspirations and dreams being forged into plans. I settled into a chair, its contours unfamiliar yet oddly comforting, and listened intently as the instructor began to outline the journey we were about to embark on together.

As days turned into nights, and presentations blended into hands-on exercises, I absorbed every detail, every strategy they laid before us. My notepad filled with scribbled thoughts and considerations, diagrams mapping out the pathway from where I stood to where I intended to be—owner of my destiny, captain of a ship sailing into commercial waters.

In the quiet moments between sessions, my phone became the lifeline to my future. Dialing numbers with practiced ease, I reached out to those who knew the terrain of my hometown market best—the current store owners. Their voices, rich with Midwestern accents, painted a picture of community and potential, lending substance to my hopes.

"Ricky-Bobby?" I asked when his familiar drawl answered the call.

"Speaking," he confirmed, a warmth in his tone that bridged the distance between San Diego and Ohio.

"Word around is you might be looking to pass the torch?" I ventured, the question hanging between us like a thread waiting to be woven into the fabric of my next chapter.

"Could be," he admitted, a note of contemplation threading through his words. "You interested?"

"More than you can imagine," I responded, not just with the intention of business but with the conviction of a man who has peered over the edge of uncertainty and chosen to leap.

Negotiations unfolded like a dance, steps measured and courteous under the watchful eye of the franchise headquarters. We spoke of numbers and timing, of visions for continuity and change. And through it all, I sensed the dawning of mutual respect, an understanding that this transaction was more than just commerce—it was legacy, it was livelihood, it was life rising anew from the ashes of trials endured.

Each night, as I lay in my hotel bed staring at the ceiling, I allowed myself to dream. Dreams of storefronts and patrons, of success built not on chance but on the indomitable will of a man forged in adversity. The days ahead shimmered with promise, a kaleidoscope of what-might-be that fueled my resolve.

"Here's to the trail blazed by persistence," I whispered into the darkness, a silent vow to honor every lesson learned, every scar earned. The path ahead was mine to tread, and I would walk it with my head held high and hope burning bright as a guiding star in the firmament of my own making. My training in San Diego now complete, it was time to get back to El Paso so that we may begin our journey back home to Ohio.

The morning came early, a soft golden hue spilling across the El Paso skyline as Shelly and I prepared to set out on our journey home. The U-Haul's engine rumbled to life with a comforting purr, a reassuring sound that spoke of reliability and the long road ahead. Attached behind it, the trailer cradled the Cadillac, a gleaming symbol of the new life awaiting us—a life I had fought for, tooth and nail.

A glance in the rearview mirror revealed Wags, the three-legged Dachshund mix we'd adopted. She was an embodiment of resilience, her one less limb not diminishing her zest for life but rather amplifying it. Her presence in the back of the Prius, along with our first dog, Mandy, nestled among blankets with Shelly at the wheel, added a sense of completeness to our caravan. We were a convoy of hope, each of us marked by life's trials, yet unyielding in our pursuit of happiness.

The roads stretched out before us like ribbons of possibility, and as we headed east, the miles unfurled one after another, carrying us toward Ohio—toward home. Landscapes changed from the coastal cliffs to arid deserts, and then to the verdant plains that signified we were nearing our destination. Each passing mile marker was a quiet victory, a testament to the distance we'd traveled, both literally and figuratively.

Our conversations through hands-free calls were sparse, punctuated by updates on traffic and rest stops, but brimming with an unspoken understanding. We were moving forward, not just geographically but in our very souls. The solitude of the drive allowed for reflection, for the appreciation of the fortitude that had carried us through darker times.

And so when the familiar skyline of our hometown finally came into view three days later, my heart swelled with a potent mixture of nostalgia and anticipation. The factories and fields, the small-town diners, and the corner stores—they all whispered of roots and beginnings. I felt the weight of history, the collective breaths of generations that had called this place home, imprinting their lives upon its canvas.

We pulled into our driveway, the gravel crunching beneath tires as if applauding our return. Stepping out of the U-Haul, I stretched and breathed in the air that seemed tinged with the scent of opportunity. Shelly opened the door of her Prius, and our dogs bounded out, eager to explore this new territory that promised stability and love.

"Welcome home," Shelly said, her smile reflecting the hope that danced in her eyes.

"Home," I echoed, feeling the word settle into my bones.

I looked around, taking in the sight of our modest house, the trees that stood like sentinels along the street, and the neighborhood that held memories yet to be made. This was more than just a geographic location—it was the starting line of a future crafted by perseverance by an unwavering belief that after every storm comes calm.

As I unloaded our belongings, each box and piece of furniture seemed to carry with it a story of survival and transformation. With each item placed within the walls of our home, I was building more than just a living space—I was crafting a sanctuary of hope, a tangible reminder that no matter what life throws your way, you can always begin anew.

"Here's to fresh starts," I murmured, not just to myself or to Shelly but to the universe that had watched me rise and fall and rise again. The sun dipped low, painting the horizon in hues of triumph, and I knew, deep in my core, that the best was yet to come.

CHAPTER 15

BETRAYAL IN BUSINESS

The moment I shook Ricky-Bobby's hand on the deal, a shiver ran up my spine. It wasn't the brisk Ohio air or a sense of foreboding; it was pure, unadulterated excitement. Here I was, about to take the reins of my very own store, a dream turning into reality right before my eyes. In that instant, I should have seen the signs. Ricky-Bobby's paranoia about government agencies and his outlandish theories on tax conspiracies were more than just eccentricities—they were glaring red flags.

"Listen, Bobby," he began, his eyes darting around as if invisible agents were lurking in every corner, "we have to keep this between us, all right? The full price can't go on the books. You know how these bloodsuckers are."

I nodded, perhaps too eagerly. The idea of owning a store was blinding, and in its luminous glow, my judgment wavered. A side loan, he said, an additional $150,000 that would flow directly from my pocket to his, circumventing the prying eyes of anyone who might question the transaction. His reasoning seemed sound at the time—a way to save on taxes, keep the ship steady. I bought into it without a second thought.

"Trust me, it's better for both of us this way," he assured me, a sly smile creeping across his face.

As days turned into weeks, and the initial thrill ebbed away, replaced by the steady rhythm of running the business, it became increasingly clear. The numbers didn't add up. The whispers of intuition that I had pushed aside now roared in my ears. The store, its value inflated by Ricky-Bobby's slick words, was never worth what he claimed. Headquarters, with their sharp pencils and sharper scrutiny, would never have sanctioned such a deal.

The payments I made to him each month weighed heavily on me, a financial albatross that I had willingly placed around my neck. Yet despite the deception, the gnawing regret, there was something else—a spark of hope, a belief in the resilience that had carried me through life's trials thus far. This was but another challenge, another test of my resolve.

I took a deep breath, feeling the crispness fill my lungs, steeling myself against the doubts and fears. My journey hadn't been easy, yet here I was, standing in my own store, the master of my destiny. Every setback was a lesson, every obstacle an opportunity to grow stronger.

With a renewed sense of purpose, I began to plan. The deceptive beginnings would not define this venture. Instead, it would be shaped by determination, ingenuity, and the unwavering belief that luck favors the bold. Ricky-Bobby's shadowy dealings would not dampen the fire within me. I would rise, as I always had, ready to prove that even from the rockiest soil, success could bloom.

The morning sun cast a hopeful glow on the weathered storefront as I approached, the keys to my future weighing heavy in my pocket. The faded sign that hung above the door was a stark reminder of the seven years this place had stood—seven years of potential stifled by mismanagement and neglect. But as I slid the key into the lock, I felt the first stirrings of ownership coursing through me. This was my ship now, and I was determined to steer it to prosperity.

Inside, the air was stale with the scent of old paper and lost opportunities. Dust motes danced in the shafts of light piercing through the blinds, illuminating the empty shelves and barren counters. It was a blank canvas, and with each step across the creaking floorboards, my mind buzzed with ideas for revitalization.

I found solace in the solitude of the space, embracing the quiet as a companion in these critical moments of introspection. Here, in the heart of Ohio, my resilience would be tested once more. Like the industrious pioneers who settled this land before me, I would cultivate success from the fallow ground.

My last week of training in Pepper Pike had been an intense whirlwind, a crash course in reality that sharpened my focus. Each day brought new insights, honing skills I didn't even know I needed until now. As Friday drew to a close, and the mentorship ended, I realized there was no template for the challenges ahead—only the relentless pursuit of improvement.

The meeting with Ricky-Bobby was brief, his demeanor evasive as always. He handed over the keys with a nonchalant flick of his wrist, offering no parting wisdom or supportive words. It mattered little; his conspiracy-laden cautionary tales and tax evasion strategies were of no use to me now. I was carving my path, one grounded in honesty and hard work.

Grateful for the solitude, I set to work clearing out the clutter from the back office, my thoughts focused on what needed to be done. It didn't take long; Ricky-Bobby had always been one for minimalism.

With the space cleared, I sat at the desk and pulled out my notebook, rereading notes and ideas from my training. I had a lot of work ahead of me, but with determination and a solid plan, I knew it was possible to turn this store around.

But then reality struck as I remembered Ricky-Bobby's parting words. No employees? That meant I would have to handle everything myself until I could find replacements. It seemed like an insurmountable task, but I refused to let doubt creep in. Instead, I focused on the potential of this place and my own abilities.

Alone, I began moving in furniture, arranging chairs and desks in a way that spoke of community and collaboration. With each piece set down, the echo of emptiness waned, replaced by the burgeoning promise of life and commerce. This wasn't just about selling products or services; it was about creating a hub where people could come together, share stories, and leave a little happier than when they arrived.

I spent the rest of the day familiarizing myself with inventory and trying to make sense of Ricky-Bobby's chaotic system. It was clear that organization was not his strong suit. But as I worked, ideas began to form in my mind—ways to streamline processes and make things more efficient.

As night fell and exhaustion set in, I locked up the store and headed home with a sense of satisfaction. This was just day one, but it felt like a small victory already.

"Ricky-Bobby may have sold me a lemon," I whispered to the empty room, "but I'll make lemonade." It was a promise to myself, a vow to turn this situation around. There was work to be done, improvements to be made, and a vision to be realized. The road ahead was uncertain, fraught with challenges, but I was no stranger to hard work or adversity.

Over the next few days and weeks, as I juggled tasks that would normally be split between multiple employees, it became clear just how much work this store needed. The shelves were emptying too quickly—a sign that restocking hadn't been happening regularly—and there were customers who stopped coming because they couldn't find what they needed.

But through it all, even when fatigue threatened to overwhelm me, I remained optimistic. This was my chance to prove myself—to show that success could be achieved without resorting to shady dealings or cutting corners.

And slowly but surely, things began to improve. With each passing day, I gained more knowledge about the business, and customers began to notice the improvements, especially the free coffee that I now provided every day.

Despite the unspoken challenges, a sense of optimism took root within me. I envisioned customers walking through the door, greeted by a vibrant atmosphere, a place that reflected the pride and dedication I intended to pour into every transaction.

With a renewed sense of purpose, I began to plan. The deceptive beginnings would not define this venture. Instead, it would be shaped by determination, ingenuity, and the unwavering belief that luck favors the bold. Ricky-Bobby's shadowy dealings would not dampen the fire within me. I would rise, as I always had, ready to prove that even from the rockiest soil, success could bloom.

The echo of the closing door reverberated through the empty space as I clutched the cold metal keys in my palm. Ricky-Bobby's final words, a nonchalant confession that the promised employees had quit, hung in the air like an ominous fog. I was alone, the weight of this new venture pressing down on me with a gravity I hadn't anticipated.

"Out of the frying pan and into the fire," I muttered to myself, a wry smile tugging at the corners of my mouth despite the fluttering panic in my chest. It would have been easy, right then, to succumb to despair—to see this not as a beginning but an end. But I've never been one to back down from a challenge. My life had been a testament to tenacity, a series of battles fought and won, often by sheer force of will.

I took a deep breath, the scent of cardboard and dust filling my nostrils grounding me. Doubt sidled up next to me, whispering seductively about defeat and impossibility. But as always, it was hope that spoke louder, that told me this, too, shall be conquered.

With no one to guide me, I became both student and teacher, learning the ropes that bound this business together. My fingers danced over the register keys, my eyes scanning item codes, absorbing everything with the urgency of a sponge in water. And when questions arose, like dragons threatening my kingdom of cardboard boxes and office supplies, I wielded my phone like a sword, cutting through uncertainty with each call for help.

Admittedly, in those early days, insecurity wrapped its tendrils around my judgment. The fear of failure, of not being enough on my own, drove me to hire more hands than necessary. Staff bustled in and out, a carousel of faces offering temporary reprieve for my aching spine, which protested the long hours and physical toll of my determination. Each evening, as I locked up and turned off the lights, I could hear the silent reproach of vertebrae worn from years of service, both to country and ambition.

But there is relief in realizing one's limits, in understanding that it's okay to lean on others sometimes. The store buzzed with activity, a hive of productivity that pulsed with the energy of shared purpose. And though my body cried out for rest, my spirit soared with every sale, every satisfied customer, every small victory that whispered, "You're doing it."

This was more than a job; it was a testament to willpower. My fledgling business was not just a reflection of me but also of the community that walked through its doors, seeking solutions, connections, a piece of the world outside their own. They didn't know the story behind the man who packaged their parcels or managed their mail. They saw only the results—a smoothly run operation, a friendly nod, resilience incarnate in the form of a neighborhood store.

In those moments of solitude, with the soft hum of fluorescent lights as my company, I'd look to the future with the optimism of a dreamer. Each package sent out was a carrier pigeon of hope, delivering messages of perseverance and possibility.

"Your move, fate," I whispered into the stillness, a grin spreading across my face. I was ready. Ready to prove that luck, indeed, favors the bold—and the determined.

*****

The morning sun filtered through the glass storefront as I flipped the sign to "Open." The scent of fresh cardboard and packing tape mingled with the rich aroma of coffee from the café next door, a comforting blend that had become my new normal. My spine ached in anticipation of the long hours ahead, but my resolve was steadfast; this store was my proving ground.

As I arranged the counter displays, a notification pinged on my phone—a Facebook post caught my eye. Allison, an old friend from high school, her words a silent plea for employment. I remembered her kind heart, her laughter echoing down the corridors of our youth. Life hadn't been easy for Allison, raising Geneva, her special-needs daughter, on her own. They were a duo of undeniable strength, and the thought of them struggling tightened something in my chest.

"Need a hand?" The message I sent was simple, but it held the weight of an opportunity, both for Allison and for me. Within days, she began working at the store, her presence a balm to the frenetic pace of commerce. She was quick to learn, quicker to smile, even when the cash register spat out receipts like a petulant child.

Geneva would sometimes accompany her mother, a sprite of a girl with a knack for organizing shelves and brightening rooms. She handled merchandise with care that belied her young years, her laughter a melody amid the cacophony of printers and phones. Geneva became an unexpected asset, her joy infectious, her work ethic mirroring her mother's.

Yet life is a river, its current relentless, and change the only constant. As seasons shifted and leaves turned, so too did Allison's path veer away from the store. Tennessee called to her, whispered promises of a fresh start, a chance at love and stability for her and Geneva. I watched them go with a mix of emotions, pride and sadness intermingled.

Their departure left a void, not just in staffing but in spirit. Their absence was palpable, a silent space where once there had been warmth and laughter. Yet their story served as a reminder—there is always hope on the horizon, always another chapter waiting to be written.

I tucked that lesson close to my heart as I faced each day, each challenge. The hum of the store became my soundtrack, the rhythm of resilience my dance. Alone again, save for the memory of friends who'd graced my journey, I leaned into the solitude.

"Here's to new beginnings," I murmured to the empty room, the echo of my voice a testament to possibility. Allison and Geneva were crafting their happiness elsewhere, while I continued to forge mine here, one package, one customer, one day at a time.

With every box I taped shut, every stamp I affixed, I sealed within them a sliver of hope. Perhaps it was luck, perhaps it was fate, or maybe it was simply the stubborn persistence of a dreamer refusing to yield. Whatever it was, it carried me forward, through pain, doubt, and fear, toward a future I was determined to shape with my own hands.

"Your move, world," I said to no one in particular, a playful defiance lighting my eyes. "I'm still standing."

The first light of dawn crept through the glass storefront, casting a glow on the faded linoleum as I stood alone among the aisles, my thoughts a swirling maelstrom. Despite the quiet, a sense of purpose pulsed within these walls, an energy born of relentless determination and hard-won victories. I had rolled up my sleeves and dug deep into the marrow of this business, reinvigorating operations like a doctor reviving a patient long-neglected.

"Let's see what we've got for today," I muttered to myself as I booted up the computer. The screen flickered to life, revealing the updated software interface—a victory in itself. Gone were the days of clunky systems that moved with the speed of molasses. This was the digital age, and my store would not be left behind.

I could still hear Allison's laughter mingled with Geneva's gentle voice, a bittersweet symphony that echoed in the now-quiet corners. Their absence was felt, but their spirit of perseverance lingered. In their honor, I had added new services, from custom packaging options to express shipping, and the community responded with open wallets and grateful smiles.

The printer hummed to life, churning out reports of increased sales—nearly 40 percent over last year. A feat, some might say, akin to turning water into wine. But beneath the sheen of success lay a stark reality: the weight of the side loan bore down on me, a relentless gravity that threatened to pull everything under. Too many employees, too many hours, and the numbers on the balance sheet began to blur, dancing a sinister tango that whispered of impending doom.

"Stay the course," I coached myself, "fix what you can each day."

And then, just when routine had begun to feel like stability, came the tremor that would send cracks spidering across the foundation I had so painstakingly laid. It was subtle at first, the arrival of the franchise representatives, their clipboards clutched like shields, their eyes scanning for inconsistencies, for failings.

My gaze fell upon the American flag that adorned the back wall, its stars and stripes a silent testament to the years I had served, to the sacrifices made. It wasn't merely fabric and color; it was a piece of my soul stitched into the history of this land, a reminder of who I was and what I had endured.

"Every inch of this place tells a story," I whispered, brushing my fingertips against the cool fabric. The flag had been my anchor, grounding me in the tumultuous seas of entrepreneurship. To the representatives, it might have been an anomaly, a decoration out of step with corporate uniformity. To me, it was a symbol of resilience, a banner under which I fought my daily battles and had literally broken my back for.

In the solitude of the morning, with invoices stacked like soldiers ready for roll call and the aroma of freshly brewed coffee hanging in the air, I fortified myself for whatever lay ahead. The store was more than a collection of shelves and merchandise; it was a living, breathing entity that bore my imprint, my sweat, and my dreams.

"Another day, another chance," I said, steeling myself with a resolve that had become my armor. The sun climbed higher, casting light on the path I had chosen, one fraught with uncertainty but rich with the promise of triumph. With every challenge faced, with every setback weathered, I grew stronger, more adept at navigating the unpredictable terrain of fate.

"Bring it on," I dared the day, a smile tugging at the edges of my lips. For I knew, deep in my bones, that luck was what happened when preparation met opportunity. And I was nothing if not prepared.

The fluorescent lights hummed above as I ran a dust cloth over the counter, my thoughts as scattered as the receipts I'd yet to file. A glance at the American flag on the wall steadied me—the same one presented to me with military honors, its colors vibrant against the sterile backdrop of the store. It was more than fabric and thread; it was my service, my sacrifice, emblematic of the perseverance that had carried me thus far.

As if on cue, the door chimed, heralding the arrival of two representatives from headquarters. Their eyes immediately locked onto Old Glory, and their lips pursed with disapproval. "You have to take that down," one of them said, gesturing toward the flag. His tone was clinical, devoid of understanding. I straightened up, my spine reminding me of the cost of that banner.

"I'm sorry, but that is the flag I was given for serving this country, and I literally broke my back to earn it," I replied, my voice calm but resolute. "The flag will remain right where it is." Their insistence was met with my unwavering stance. I demanded a court order that they could not produce. They left, defeated. The flag stayed. My customers never voiced a complaint—in fact, many shared nods of respect when they passed by it.

About a month later, the chime of the phone broke the rhythm of my morning routine. It was Mark, my biggest account, responsible for keeping the lights on and the water running. Unease crept in as he relayed his encounter with company sales reps, their visit to his office unexpected, their offers too good to be true. "What are the rates?" I asked, sinking into my chair as though bracing for impact. He rattled off numbers that sounded eerily familiar—because they were my numbers. The very rates I paid as a franchisee. A cold realization settled in my stomach; headquarters had just stolen $3,000 monthly from me.

Betrayal snaked through my veins, hot and poisonous. "Bastards," I muttered once the line went dead, staring blankly at the wall. There hung the flag, undisturbed, its stars and stripes a stark contrast to the shadow that now loomed over my business.

Yet even as anger threatened to consume me, I felt the embers of hope stir within. This flag had witnessed battles before, both mine and those of my nation, enduring through strife and turmoil. The resolve that had fortified me in uniform surged anew. No, I would not surrender to despair. I would fight, adapt, survive. For under that flag, I had sworn an oath—not only to my country but to myself—to press on, to rise above, to overcome. And so I would, one day at a time, one challenge at a time. My grip tightened on the edge of the desk, determination setting my jaw. "Bring it on," I whispered to the empty room, the echo a quiet battle cry. Fortune had dealt me a harsh hand, but luck? Luck was still mine to command.

The phone was like a lead weight in my hand. My fingers, normally steady from years of military discipline, trembled ever so slightly as I dialed the number for headquarters. This kind of treachery wasn't just business; it was personal. They had gone behind my back, undercut me in the most underhanded way possible, shaking the very foundation of trust that is supposed to exist between a franchisee and their parent company. "Hello, this is Bobby Quayle. We need to talk about my customer—the one you've just offered my rates to," I said, my voice taut with barely restrained fury.

The silence on the other end was pregnant with unease. "Mr. Quayle, we assure you it wasn't intentional," came the eventual reply, muffled and hesitant. "And we promise it won't happen again."

"Your 'assurances' don't pay my bills or cover what you've poached from me." The franchise agreement was clear, and I made sure to remind them of that. "You know full well this is against our terms."

"We understand your frustration, but unfortunately, there's nothing we can do about the offer extended to your customer."

"Unbelievable," I snapped before ending the call, the taste of betrayal souring my mouth.

As the hours waned into evening, Shelly listened quietly while I recounted the day's ordeal. Her presence was a steady beacon, her eyes reflecting the storm of emotions roiling within me. "Maybe selling is your best option," she gently suggested, her voice a soothing counterpoint to the chaos in my mind. To sell would be to admit defeat, to let go of the dream and effort poured into every corner of the store. It would mean turning my back on the staff who had become family, on the community that had started to rely on us. Yet Shelly's words lingered, haunting in their pragmatism. I gazed at the flag, its fabric whispering tales of perseverance and valor. No, I was not ready to fold. Not when there was still fight left in me. Not when the emblem of my service, of our nation's resilience, hung proudly on my wall. This was but another trial, a test of fortitude. "Thank you," I said to Shelly, squeezing her hand, gratitude mingling with renewed determination. "But I'm not giving up. Not yet."

That night, the stars outside seemed to wink knowingly, as if they, too, understood the value of holding on just a little bit longer. In their celestial dance, I saw the reflection of my own journey—a tapestry of challenges met and conquered. Tomorrow, I'd face this new battle head-on, armed with the knowledge that even the darkest moments could be transformed into opportunities. For now, though, I held onto hope, letting it anchor me until the dawn.

The morning sun peeked through the blinds, falling across the ledger strewn with figures and calculations. I had been up since the crack of dawn, poring over every expense, weighing the cost of loyalty against the harsh reality of survival. My fingers tapped a steady rhythm on the desktop, echoing the beat of my racing heart. I knew what had to be done. "Shelly," I said, glancing at my wife who sat at the kitchen table sipping her coffee, "I've got to let some people go today."

She set down her cup with a soft clink, her eyes searching mine for the resolve she knew was warring with regret within me. "You're doing what's necessary, Bobby," she reassured me, her voice steady and her hand reaching out to still mine. "They'll understand."

With each name that I circled on the employee roster, a part of me felt like I was severing a lifeline, not just for them but for myself as well. It wasn't just about cutting costs; it was about preserving hope, keeping the dream alive, even if it meant downsizing to the bare bones. As I prepared for the day ahead, the phone rang—the ringtone I had assigned for business opportunities. It was the organizer of the sports collectibles event, his voice brimming with enthusiasm. "We want you there, Bobby. Your store has the reputation for reliability, and we need someone to handle the shipping for all the purchases."

A flicker of excitement ignited in my chest. This could be it, the break we needed. I jumped on the opportunity, gathering every resource left at my disposal. Marketing the event became my sole focus, a beacon in the fog of financial uncertainty. The event was a whirlwind of activity. Collectors and enthusiasts bustled about, eager hands exchanging treasures and wallets opening wide. Our shipping booth was swamped, a line snaking around the corner as customers entrusted us with their prized possessions. The register chimed steadily, and with each transaction, a weight lifted from my shoulders.

"Looks like we hit the jackpot, huh?" Shelly whispered to me as we tallied up the week's earnings. It was more than we'd made in two months, a staggering sum that would cover the pressing debts and keep us afloat for a little while longer. I wrapped an arm around her, allowing myself a moment of relief.

"Thank goodness," I murmured, the words a silent prayer of gratitude. But even in the midst of this small victory, reality loomed on the horizon. Payday approached, and with the influx of cash came the hard decisions. Some of the employees would receive their last paycheck from me. They depended on this job, and in turn, I depended on their hard work and dedication. It pained me to think of the impact this would have on their lives.

The evening before payday, I took a long walk, my steps carrying me past the homes of the very people who would feel the sting of my choices. I rehearsed the conversations in my mind, each word heavy with the burden of leadership and the cost of dreams deferred. "Tomorrow," I promised myself, looking up at the stars that mirrored the spark of hope still burning within me, "I'll start anew. We'll build back up, piece by piece." And with that thought cradling my resolve, I turned back home, ready to face whatever the next day would bring.

As I locked the door to the store that evening, I couldn't help but pause for a moment, leaning against the cool metal and taking in a deep breath. The weight of my decisions laid heavy on my shoulders, yet there was a spark of hope that refused to be extinguished. Valarie and Zach were inside, finishing up for the day, and I thought about their contributions to the store's survival.

Valarie's laughter filtered through the glass, her voice like a beacon of normalcy amid the chaos. She had transitioned from the bank to my store with such grace, trading the relentless pursuit of quotas for the sincere customer service we offered. I could still remember her first day, how she organized the books with meticulous care, a skill honed from years behind the counter at the bank. Her presence brought stability to our operations, and her easy smile made even the longest days bearable. I knew that parting ways with any employee would affect her deeply; she had become not just a manager but a friend to all who worked here.

Turning away from the door, I watched as Zach carefully stacked boxes, his movements practiced and efficient. The young man had grown so much since he started—no longer the aimless soul who hung around the wrong crowds but a dependable and skilled worker. His father had been right to believe that a change of scenery could reroute his path. Zach's transformation was one of the silent victories in my life, a testament to the power of second chances. Together, we had faced shipments and inventory challenges, each hurdle surmounted strengthening the bond between us. He was proof that even the most wayward journey could find direction.

As I walked toward my car, I let the quiet of the evening wash over me. Tomorrow would bring difficult conversations, but tonight, I chose to focus on the good. We had weathered storms before, and resilience was etched into the very foundation of this business. With Valarie's tenacity and Zach's newfound purpose, we created more than just a place of commerce; it was a haven where lost souls found grounding, and weary hearts found ease.

"Tomorrow," I whispered to myself, "we face what comes with heads held high, because today, we've proven just how much we can achieve." The stars above seemed to twinkle in agreement, their light a gentle reminder that darkness eventually gives way to dawn. And with that reassurance cradling my spirit, I drove home, ready to rebuild, ready to inspire, and above all, ready to hope.

The sun was still climbing when I pulled into the familiar space behind the store, its rays casting a warm glow on the concrete. Today was payday—a day of obligation and satisfaction, where I could tangibly reward the hard work of Valarie and Zach. With the successful sports collectibles event fresh in my memory, I felt a quiet confidence as I locked my car and made a mental note to hit the shooting range later, the weight of my Glock 9mm an afterthought in the trunk.

Pushing through the back door, the familiar scent of cardboard and ink greeted me, a scent that had become synonymous with the daily grind and small victories. I nodded to Valarie, who was already deep in her morning routine, her focus unshaken. Zach was there, too, humming softly as he organized the counter, his movements more assured than when he first started. They were my anchors in the choppy seas of retail, their presence a constant reminder that together, we could weather any storm.

Settling into my chair, I powered up the computer, the familiar chime signaling the start of another busy day. Today, I would reinforce their trust, pay them for their efforts, and maybe even share some good news about the uptick in sales. The screen flickered to life, and I navigated to the banking portal, anticipation tinged with the formality of the task at hand.

That's when the numbers, or lack thereof, hit me like a rogue wave—my account balance glaring back with a stark, unforgiving zero. Disbelief clawed at my chest as I scanned for some mistake, some clerical error that could explain this catastrophe. But the harsh truth bore down upon me; headquarters had taken everything. Every dollar from the event that had promised respite and recovery snatched away without warning.

My hands trembled on the keyboard, a bitter cocktail of shock and anger coursing through me. I leaned back in the chair, squinting at the screen as if by sheer willpower I could conjure the missing funds from the digital ether. It was supposed to be a day of celebration, of rewards earned, and instead, it was a nightmare scenario unfolding in broad daylight.

"Everything okay, boss?" Zach's voice cut through my daze, his concern palpable.

I managed a tight smile, not trusting my voice just yet. "Just a little hiccup, I'm on it," I lied, unwilling to cast a shadow over their morning. This wasn't their burden to bear—not yet. I needed to think, to plan, to strategize. If resilience had taught me anything, it was that hope was never truly lost, only momentarily obscured.

"Keep things running, I'll be right back," I told them, standing with a purpose I didn't feel. As I stepped out the back door, the sunlight seemed to mock me, but I shook off the despair. Over the years, I'd learned that luck is often disguised as misfortune, and every setback carried the seed of a new beginning.

Today would not be defined by a number on a screen but by the resolve to rise above it. For Valarie, for Zach, for all those who depended on the haven we'd created, I would find a way through. The road ahead was uncertain, but one thing was crystal clear: I wouldn't let this defeat us. Not now, not ever.

I returned to the store and I grabbed my coat with hands that trembled, not from the chill of the air-conditioned store but from a storm of anxiety that raged within. The murmurs of the staff behind me felt distant as I pushed through the glass door, stepping into a world that seemed to have shifted on its axis. With every step toward my car, my mind raced faster than my feet could carry me.

"Got some things to take care of," I said over my shoulder, hoping my voice didn't betray the turmoil inside. They nodded, their faces a blend of curiosity and concern, but they were used to me handling things—fires, they'd call them. Little did they know this was a blaze I wasn't sure I could extinguish.

The drive to the Metroparks felt automatic, muscle memory guiding me while my thoughts spiraled. How to explain this? How to keep their faith when mine was faltering? My employees were more than just names on a payroll; they were family, friends, lives intertwined with the heartbeat of the business we built together.

As I parked by the familiar trails, the serenity of the park enveloped me like a comforting embrace. The trees stood tall and resilient, weathering storms and seasons, much like I've done throughout my life. I needed their wisdom now, their silent strength.

Stride by stride along the paved path, the rhythms of nature began to work their subtle magic. Chipmunks scampered across roots, undeterred by obstacles. Birds sang melodies of persistence. The emerald canopy above whispered promises of renewal and growth. The Metroparks, my sanctuary, reminded me that even the mightiest oak grew from the smallest acorn.

I had been here before—not this path, perhaps, but this precipice between despair and determination. Doubt had been a frequent visitor in my life, but each time it knocked, I answered with tenacity. This wouldn't be any different. I couldn't let it be.

My heart pounds in my chest like a sledgehammer as I frantically search for a way out of this mess. My mind races, trying to come up with solutions, but they seem to slip away like wispy clouds on a windy day. Sweat beads on my forehead as I contemplate desperate measures—deferring payments, offering discounts, hosting an emergency sale.

Time becomes irrelevant as I wander deeper and deeper into the Metroparks, the weight of my problems pressing down on me until it feels like I'm suffocating. I shut off my phone, unable to face the barrage of concerned calls and messages from my family and employees.

With each step, my depression deepens, engulfing me like a thick black cloud. Self-doubt consumes me as I berate myself for every mistake—the bad deal with the previous owner, over-hiring employees, and even being patriotic in defiance of headquarters at my own expense.

The forest becomes a physical manifestation of my despair as I lose myself in its depths. How could I have been so foolish? The realization hits me like a punch in the gut, and I can't shake the feeling that I am nothing but a failure.

And as the darkness closes in around me, I realize that this may be where I will spend the rest of my days—lost and alone in an endless forest of failures.

CHAPTER 16

A MOMENT OF DESPAIR

The verdant embrace of the Metroparks had always been a sanctuary for me, a place where whispers of nature could hush the clamor of my thoughts. Yet today, as I ventured deeper into its heart, those whispers fell silent, swallowed by an unsettling stillness. My footsteps on the forest floor were soft and methodical, each one taking me further from the world I knew—a world that, at this moment, seemed a distant memory.

Before I had set out on this impromptu trek, a prickling sense of forethought compelled me to visit the trunk of my car. It was there, resting atop a clutter of tools and emergency supplies, that my Glock 9mm lay in wait—my companion for the range session I had planned later. Its familiar weight in my hands was a stark reminder of the cautionary life I led, always prepared, always wary. Securing it in my waistband, I pressed on into the embrace of the woods.

The hours slipped by unnoticed, as if time itself grew weary of keeping pace with my wandering. It had been eight hours since I left the store, eight hours since my routine life had unraveled into this silent odyssey. With each passing minute, the concern from my coworkers and Shelly would have magnified, their voices piling up unheard on my voicemail like leaves in autumn.

Shelly, ever vigilant, must have felt that first twinge of panic when she saw the empty space where the Glock usually rested. I could almost hear the tremble in her voice as she dialed the police, her fear painting the worst pictures in the void of my absence. The issuance of an APB was a testament to the gravity of my disappearance—an echo of distress rippling through the community.

But here, amid towering oaks and whispering pines, the search parties and sirens couldn't reach me. I became an island, isolated in a sea of greenery, disconnected from the chaos of civilization. No traffic hummed in the distance; no chatter of people disturbed the serenity. It was just me, Bobby Quayle, alone with the earth and sky.

My mind, that relentless machine, churned with thoughts both dark and light. Resilience is not a stranger to me; I've tasted the bitterness of adversity and spat it out with defiance. Hope, that elusive bird, often perched upon my shoulder, even when the clouds loomed heavy. And luck? Well, some say you make your own luck—I say it's a dance with fate you learn step by step.

In the depths of the Metroparks, under the canopy of ancient trees, I clung to those ideals: resilience, hope, and luck. They were threads woven into the fabric of my being, and though frayed, they held. With every breath of forest air, I sought to stitch them tighter, to patch the worn places in my spirit. This was not the end of my story—it was merely a page turned, waiting for the ink to dry.

The weasel moved with a grace that seemed almost otherworldly, its sleek form undulating like liquid through the dense foliage along the riverbank. I watched, mesmerized by its single-minded pursuit of sustenance, as it deftly plucked crayfish from the shallows. There was an elegance to survival in nature, a stark contrast to the chaos of human existence.

Perched on a rock, I felt the weight of the Glock against my side—a cold, metallic reminder of the range visit that never happened. In front of me, the rhythmic motion of the weasel's hunt played out like a dance of life and death, instigating a reflection on my own existence. Should I just end it here? The question clawed at my mind with the persistence of a raven pecking at carrion.

My marriage, once a beacon of shared dreams and laughter, was now a shipwreck caught in the relentless tide of disappointment and unmet expectations. The thought of Shelly—strong, compassionate Shelly—flitted through my consciousness. She deserved better than the shadow of a man I had become. And yet her faith in me never wavered, even when mine did.

"I have no children that count on me," another taunting whisper came. My wife will be okay in the long run. Mother, resilient as the oak trees around me, would persevere as she always had. Deb, though battling her own storms, would surely find shelter in our mother's unwavering love.

And Mandy and Wags—my loyal companions, whose boundless affection demanded so little and gave so much—they would be cherished by Shelly. They would miss me, perhaps for a time, but dogs live in the joy of the moment, not the sorrow of yesterdays or the uncertainty of tomorrows.

With a trembling hand, I withdrew the Glock from my waistband, its presence an aberration amid the symphony of nature. How long had I sat there, lost in the tumult of my soul, while shadows crept across the river like silent sentinels?

The world would just be better off without me, I mused, the dark thought swirling in my mind like leaves caught in an eddy. Yet as I held the instrument of my potential demise, I couldn't help but notice the way life thrived around me—the weasel with its catch, the dragonflies skimming the water's surface, the steadfast trees reaching for the sky.

These were entities of resilience, each embodying hope in their tenacity to endure, to grow, to exist. Could I not learn from them? Was there not some sliver of luck nestled in the folds of my despair, waiting to be uncovered?

In the stillness of the Metroparks, where civilization's cacophony was reduced to a distant memory, I found a clarity that had eluded me amid the noise. Maybe, just maybe, this wasn't the end. Maybe it was a turning point, a chance to reclaim the threads of resilience, hope, and luck that had woven the tapestry of my life thus far.

The weasel, successful in its quest, darted away with a bounty to sustain it another day. In that simple act of perseverance, I saw a mirror to my own potential path—one that led away from the brink, back toward the light.

The chill of the Glock's metal bit at my temple, a stark contrast to the warmth of my skin—an unwanted kiss from an unwelcome suitor. The weight of it seemed to anchor me to that rock, as if it were all that kept me from floating away into the ether. The scent of gunpowder, a grim reminder of past days spent honing skills I never thought I'd turn toward myself, drifted up and filled my senses. My eyes, blurred by the tears that welled within them, still caught the motionless tableau of nature around me.

I watched as the forest held its breath, the creatures suspending their dance of life. They had become spectators to my profound despair, silent witnesses to the battle raging within a man whose heart was heavy with defeat. The smallest twitch of my finger would be the crescendo to this morbid symphony. I tightened my grip, the trembling in my hands an eerie mimicry of the leaves quivering on their branches, my finger began to pull against the trigger.

Suddenly, the dense canopy above parted as if by some divine hand, allowing a shaft of blinding sunlight to break through. It was like a scene from a play, orchestrated by a higher power. The light was otherworldly, making the forest floor glow with ethereal beauty. All around me, the shadows that had been clinging to my thoughts seemed to dissipate in this holy radiance.

I felt myself being lifted up, engulfed in a sense of peace and serenity. The light was brighter than the sun yet somehow softer, as if it were coming from within rather than without. It filled me with an overwhelming warmth and joy, drowning out the darkness that had been consuming me.

And then I heard it. A beautiful song that seemed to emanate from every living thing around me. It was like nothing I had ever heard before—pure and soulful, with lyrics that spoke directly to my heart. As Carrie Underwood's "Jesus Take the Wheel" echoed through the forest, I felt as though I was being transported back in time.

Memories flooded my mind—memories of childhood adventures in Cleveland, where winters were harsh, but summers were full of wonder and joy. High school days spent with friends whose laughter still rang in my ears. The faces of loved ones who had helped shape me into the person I am today—Shelly's kind and tender gaze, Mom's unwavering love, Deb's shared struggles, Sergeant Martinez's brotherhood, Bernd's unbreakable friendship.

Each image was a reminder of battles fought and won, of resilience not yet extinguished. There were moments of joy too: the sound of Mary's laughter before our paths diverged, Mandy and Wags chasing each other in the yard with blissful abandon, and the store, a dream made real through sweat and sacrifice. These were the landmarks of my journey, the proof of life's relentless march forward—a march I was still a part of, despite the despair that clouded my vision.

In that moment, all of these memories converged, weaving together into a tapestry of gratitude and hope. And I knew then that no matter how dark things may seem, there is always light shining through—whether it be through nature or music or cherished memories. In that moment surrounded by nature's symphony and embraced by divine love, I found solace and strength to carry on.

My resolve faltered, my grip loosened, and the instrument of my potential end became nothing more than a cold, lifeless thing in my hand. I was not done here—not yet. There were still melodies to hear, still sunbeams to chase. With a heart that began to beat with the promise of tomorrow, I chose to step back from the brink and embrace the resilience that had carried me through life's trials—the same resilience I saw reflected in the natural world around me.

The haunting melody of the song ebbed and flowed, its lyrics a piercing reminder of my troubled existence. The strumming of the guitar seemed to intensify as Carrie's voice pleaded for salvation. With each note, I felt my resolve weakening until finally, as she sang the words "I'm letting go, give me one more chance…save me from this road I'm on," I couldn't bear it any longer. Tears streamed down my face as I released the gun that had been a symbol of my destructive path. It clattered against the rocky ground, its metallic clang a stark contrast to the soft murmur of the river nearby.

For a moment, everything was still as I fought against the tumultuous emotions raging within me. But then, with trembling hands and a shaky breath, I took my first step toward redemption, guided by Carrie's angelic voice and the gentle rustle of leaves in the breeze.

As the final notes of the song faded, the visions retreated, leaving me with a sense of raw exposure. But in that vulnerability lay a truth that resonated deep within my core. This moment of darkness was but a shadow cast by the many lights of my existence. To extinguish my flame now would be to deny the brightness of what had been and what could still be.

A gust of wind swept over the river, ruffling the leaves and tousling my hair as if to jolt me further from the edge of despair. I clung to the boulder, feeling it steady and unyielding beneath me. As the breeze passed, there was a softness in the air—a gentle exhale of relief from the Metroparks themselves. Nature, in her boundless empathy, seemed to wrap her arms around me, whispering assurances that life, indeed, would go on.

With legs that felt both weightless and leaden, I stood up, leaving behind the rock that had been my precipice. The setting sun cast a warm glow across Berea, painting my hometown in hues of hope. Each step toward the car felt like a mile, and my shadow stretched long across the path, a tangible reminder that even in darkness, I was not alone. The mosquitoes buzzed hungrily around me, but their biting seemed trivial now—a nuisance easily swatted away compared to the abyss I had just skirted.

Doubts began to crowd my thoughts as I navigated the dimming woodland trails. Shelly's face flashed before me, her eyes filled with concern and love—the same love that had seen us through countless trials. Would she understand this one? My employees, who relied on me for guidance and stability, how could I explain the depth of my despair to them? The fear of being judged, of being labeled "unstable" or "crazy" clawed at me with invisible talons.

Yet as I walked, I realized something vital had shifted inside me. The world hadn't changed; the store's ledgers were still awash in red, my marriage still needed mending, and there were still no children to bear my name. But I, Bobby Quayle, had veered back from oblivion. In the cool evening air, every breath became a testament to perseverance, each step a declaration that I would fight for another dawn, another chance.

"Are they all going to think I am crazy? Will they hate me?" I whispered into the growing dark. No answer came, only the rustling of leaves and the distant call of a night bird. Yet somehow, the silence wasn't empty. It hummed with the potential of what tomorrow might bring, a blank page upon which to start anew.

I had faced the darkest part of myself out there among the whispering trees and come back whole. If I could do that, surely facing those I cared about was a challenge I could meet. And no matter their reaction, I knew one thing for certain—I would not face it alone. Resilience, it seems, is not just about surviving the storm but also about having the courage to walk back into the light after the rain has ceased.

As Berea's familiar skyline drew closer, silhouetted against the twilight sky, I felt a stirring of hope. There would be consequences, yes, but also conversations, healing, and maybe, just maybe, a little bit of luck. With a heart lighter than it had been for hours, I stepped out of the forest and into the fading light of day.

The familiar crunch of gravel under my tires was a stark contrast to the softness of the forest floor I'd left behind. As I pulled into the driveway, the weight of my decision—or rather, my indecision—settled in my chest. I turned off the car, the silence amplifying the pounding of my heart as I reached for my phone. It flickered to life with a series of missed calls and messages that blurred before my eyes. I ignored them all, sending a simple text to Shelly: "I'm home."

Stepping out of the car, I felt the coolness of the garage against my skin, a stark reminder of the evening's chill. The house loomed large and empty, the usual cacophony of welcome from Mandy and Wags conspicuously absent. My hand fumbled for the light switch, the fluorescent tubes flickering hesitantly before casting their sterile glow over the space.

"Odd," I murmured, noting the absence of Shelly's car. I walked through the door connecting the garage to the kitchen, the sense of unease growing with each step. The house held its breath, waiting for me to discover what lay within its walls. I called out, but only silence greeted me.

Then the knock. Sharp, insistent—a demand rather than a request. "Mr. Quayle, this is the police department, please open the door slowly and let us see your hands."

My mind raced. *Police?* Why were they here? A cold sweat broke out across my forehead as fear took hold, gripping me with icy fingers. I moved toward the door, every muscle tensed, ready for whatever came next. With a deep breath, I opened it.

"Evening, Officers," I managed to say, voice steady despite the tremors I could feel building within me.

"Mr. Quayle, please step back and keep your hands where we can see them," one of the officers instructed firmly, yet not unkindly.

I complied, stepping into the kitchen, the center of so many warm memories now transformed into an interrogation room. One officer kept his eyes fixed on me, while the other scanned the surroundings, undoubtedly piecing together a narrative I had yet to fully understand.

"Is there something wrong, Officers?" I asked, though I suppose I already knew. Someone must have seen the Glock, perhaps drawn conclusions that weren't far from the truth.

"Your family's been worried about you, Mr. Quayle," the officer watching me replied. His words carried the weight of concern, not accusation. They saw me, not just the shell of a man who had wandered too close to the edge but someone who still mattered—to someone, at least.

Fear began to ebb, replaced by the realization that even in the depths of my despair, people had cared enough to look for me, to bring me home. Luck, it seemed, hadn't completely abandoned me.

"Let's make sure everything's all right," the same officer said, his voice softer now. "We're just here to help."

Help. That simple word echoed through the hollows of my thoughts, filling spaces I didn't realize needed filling. In that moment, standing in my own kitchen under the watchful gaze of law enforcement, I understood—resilience wasn't just bouncing back, it was accepting the hand extended to you, however unexpected the source.

"Thank you," I whispered, the gratitude catching in my throat, "I think I do need help."

And as those words left my lips, a new kind of strength began to take root—one that promised hope and hinted at redemption. This wasn't the end of my story; it was merely a difficult chapter. Tomorrow, the sun would rise again, and with it, so would I.

The officers' silhouettes formed a stark contrast against the warm glow of my kitchen lights as I stood there, the cold linoleum floor grounding me in reality. They surveyed the room, eyes eventually settling on me, worn and weary from the day's ordeal. One officer, his badge glistening dimly, spoke up.

"Mr. Quayle, where is your gun now?" he asked, his tone official yet not abrasive.

"It's in my car," I replied, my voice steadier than I felt. "I had plans to go to the range today."

"Really?" Another officer chimed in, his skepticism palpable. "I've heard that place is pretty pricey."

I met his gaze, understanding the gravity of their concern. "I wouldn't know about the cost. The owner is a client of mine, and it's a convenient stop on my way back from work," I explained, hoping my honesty would resonate with them.

Their eyes then drifted down to my muddy attire, evidence of my earlier escapade. "Your wife and friends are worried sick about you. Where have you been for the past ten hours?" they probed further.

It was the worry in their voices, the genuine fear for my well-being, that finally crumbled my defenses. Tears, unbidden, began to blur my vision as the dam of emotions broke free. "I…I almost did something irreversible today," I confessed, each word heavy with the weight of my near miss. "I thought about ending my life."

The air grew thick with my admission, the confession hanging between us like a specter. I told them of the crushing financial burden that threatened to topple the store, my dreams, my everything. The despair that had driven me to the brink, the sense of utter failure that had enveloped me in the silent woods.

As the veneer of authority fell away, I saw the change in their demeanor. Their stance softened, and the lines of duty on their faces seemed to smooth over with humanity. They understood that before them stood not a criminal but a man who had lost his footing on life's slippery slope and needed a hand to regain his balance.

"Mr. Quayle," one officer said, the edge of authority now replaced with compassion, "you're not alone in this."

In those simple words, I found an unexpected solace. A lifeline had been thrown to me, not in the form of a rescue rope but through the power of shared empathy. It was a reminder that even in our most isolated moments, connections—unseen and unspoken—bind us all.

A new resolve began to stir within me, a quiet determination fueled by the realization that I was still here, still breathing, still capable of facing another day. My story wasn't over; it was merely awaiting its next chapter, and I was the author holding the pen.

Through the mist of my tears, I glimpsed the hope that tomorrow might bring: an opportunity to rebuild, to make amends, and to prove that the resilience which had carried me this far would see me through yet again. With luck's fickle nature perhaps swayed in my favor, I prepared to step forward into the unknown, fortified by the knowledge that I wasn't taking that step alone.

The evening air was cool against my skin, a contrast to the warm concern that washed over me from the men and women in blue of Olmsted Falls. I felt the eyes of my neighborhood upon me, their gazes filled with worry rather than judgment. It's not often an ambulance arrives at your doorstep without a sense of impending tragedy.

"Mr. Quayle," Sergeant Smith said, her voice steady and firm, "we've arranged transportation to the hospital. This is for you—to get the help you need."

I nodded, the gravity of her words sinking in like stones in a still pond. "I understand," I managed to say, my voice hoarse from the tears I had shed only moments before. "Just let me grab my meds."

The officers moved with a professionalism that belied their empathy, retrieving my medications with swift efficiency. They understood the delicate balance of maintaining authority while providing support.

As I walked toward the waiting ambulance, flanked by the officers, I couldn't help but think of how their presence gave me a sense of security I hadn't felt in a long while. My footsteps were heavy, each one a reminder of the burden I bore, of the despair that had almost consumed me. Yet with each step, I also felt a growing determination to face my troubles head-on. There was hope in confrontation, strength in acknowledging weakness.

Our neighbors watched from behind curtains and over fences as I approached the ambulance. Their faces were a mosaic of concern, curiosity, and perhaps a touch of relief. Community—it had always been there, even when I felt most isolated.

"Ready, sir?" one of the paramedics asked as the back doors of the ambulance swung open.

"Ready as I'll ever be," I replied, a wry smile breaking through. I climbed into the vehicle without assistance, a small act of autonomy that signaled my willingness to embark on this new path.

The doors closed with a definitive thud, sealing me inside. I settled onto the stretcher, the crisp sheets a stark contrast to the chaos of my recent emotions. As we pulled away, I caught sight of the fading sunset through the window—a splash of colors against the sky, a promise that no matter how dark the night, the dawn would always come.

There, in the sterile confines of the ambulance, moving steadily toward help, I allowed myself to believe in the possibility of change. The road ahead would be fraught with challenges, but for the first time in what felt like an eternity, I felt equipped to meet them—not because the obstacles had lessened but because I had rediscovered an inner fortitude I thought lost.

I would rebuild, piece by piece, starting with the broken man in the back of that ambulance. And though the journey would be mine alone, the support of those around me—caring friends, concerned neighbors, a dedicated wife—served as beacons of light guiding me through the darkness. This was my road to redemption, paved not with certainty but with hope and the will to endure.

The frigid air of the emergency room was a striking contrast to the turmoil that burned within me, each breath a testament to the life I'd almost relinquished. A sterile symphony played around me— monitors beeping, nurses bustling, the distant wails of an ambulance. It was here, on a narrow gurney under the blinding glare of fluorescent lights, that I found myself shackled not by restraints but by the weight of my own despair.

A police officer stood at the threshold of my cubicle, his posture rigid with duty yet softened by a hint of empathy in his eyes. He was a silent guardian, a reminder of the reality that had nearly slipped through my fingers.

Through the curtain's slight parting, my ears caught the heated exchange between the ER doctor and someone from the VA. The doctor's voice rose, crackling with indignation, "What do you mean you don't want him? Given all the bad publicity the VA has had recently, do you really want to abandon a veteran who nearly took his own life?" His words punctuated the sterile environment like thunderclaps, stirring something deep within my chest—a mixture of sorrow and gratitude.

"Seriously? An ER is not really appropriate for his condition, wouldn't you agree?" There was a pause, a moment where hope and bureaucracy waged war on the other end of the line. Then, with a sound resonant of finality, the phone slammed down, its echo reverberating against the cold walls, mirroring the disgust that coursed through the doctor's veins.

"That doesn't surprise me at all," my voice cracked the silence, rising unbidden from a place of raw honesty. The doctor turned, his face a picture of shock and self-reproach. "Oh you heard that?" he muttered, chagrined.

"Don't worry, sir, we will get you taken care of," he stated firmly, the promise hanging in the air as he strode away, a man at odds with a system failing those it vowed to protect.

In that hollow space, amid the mechanical hums and the scent of antiseptics, I clung to his assurance like a lifeline. It was a sliver of light in the dim corridor of uncertainty—a beacon guiding me back from the abyss. I knew the road ahead would be strewn with hurdles, some perhaps higher than I could envision. But there was solace in knowing that even strangers harbored a desire to see me through this darkest hour.

I lay back, allowing the myriad thoughts to cascade through my mind. The past could not be undone; the mistakes and missteps were etched into the very fabric of who I was. Yet it was precisely those imperfections, those scars, that served as reminders of my capacity to endure, to adapt, to survive.

Hope is an audacious thing—it dares to blossom in adversity's shadow, urging fractured souls toward the promise of a new day. And as I lay there, a mosaic of vulnerability and resilience, I began to understand that hope was not just a fleeting sentiment. It was the essence of our shared humanity, the heartbeat of a world that refused to succumb to despair.

So as I awaited what the future held, I allowed myself to be introspective yet hopeful, understanding that luck often comes to those who choose to see the sunrise through the storm. Tomorrow was an unwritten page, and I, Bobby Quayle, still had a pen in hand.

The sirens' wail had long since fallen silent, yet their echo seemed to linger as the ambulance rolled steadily eastward. I lay on a stretcher, my gaze fixed on the narrow window, observing the world blurring by—a tapestry of life continuing oblivious to my own inner turmoil. Drivers in their cars glanced my way, their expressions a cocktail of curiosity and compassion. It tugged at something within me, this notion that perfect strangers could spare a thought for a man they knew nothing about.

I turned my head away, staring up at the sterile white interior of the ambulance. The paramedic had offered words of comfort earlier, but now we were both ensconced in our own reveries. Memories danced behind my eyelids—snapshots of a life fraught with challenges but also peppered with pockets of joy. Shelly's smile, the rough-and-tumble playfulness of Mandy and Wags, the camaraderie with Bernd—all of it a stark contrast to the cold steel of the gurney beneath me.

As the journey unfolded, each minute stretched into an eternity, the longest forty-five minutes of my existence. My thoughts were a whirlwind, yet amid the chaos, there was an undercurrent of serenity. Hope, that stubborn weed, sprouted in the cracked earth of my psyche. I wasn't sure what salvation would look like, but the act of being transported to help was a lifeline thrown into the tempestuous seas of my mind.

Arriving at the VA Hospital felt akin to crossing some unseen threshold. A police officer stood sentinel outside the vehicle, his uniform a beacon of order in my disheveled world. He escorted me with a quiet professionalism to "the Tower"—a moniker that held ominous undertones, evoking images of isolation and despair. Yet as we traversed the halls, I reminded myself that this was not a prison but a refuge where healing could begin.

The night that followed was punctuated by the cacophony of troubled souls. Shouts and sobs permeated the walls, each cry a reminder of shared suffering. Sleep proved elusive, a fleeting visitor that brushed past me but never settled. Fatigue gnawed at my bones, but even in the midst of this nocturnal symphony, I clung to a sense of hopeful anticipation.

There was a peculiar kinship in this place—an unspoken bond among those who wrestled with their inner demons. In the echoing cries, I heard not just distress but the resilience of the human spirit, fighting to reclaim itself from the clutches of darkness. It was this collective strength that buoyed me, reaffirming my belief that tomorrow could be kinder than today.

As dawn's first light began to seep through the barred windows, I reflected on the journey that had led me here. The path ahead was shrouded in uncertainty, but there was solace in knowing that I was not alone. The very fact that I was here, breathing, thinking, feeling—that in itself was a victory, however small.

In the end, life is not just the sum of our triumphs but also the grace with which we navigate our defeats. And so as I awaited the coming day, weary yet undefeated, I embraced the promise of a new beginning. Luck, after all, has a way of finding those who have the courage to bet on the dawn after the longest of nights.

Stepping through the threshold of the day room, I felt as though I had entered a theater where each actor was lost in their own tragic play. Some were pacing with frantic energy, others sat in corner seats muttering to unseen companions. A man repeatedly thumped his forehead against the pale green wall, as if trying to awaken from a nightmare that held him captive. The cacophony of voices, both real

and imagined, created a chaotic symphony, which somehow under-
scored the profound silence of personal despair.

I found myself an unoccupied chair by the window, the vinyl
cool and unwelcoming beneath me. My gaze drifted across the room,
taking in the spectacle of suffering and survival. It was like witnessing
a carousel of souls, each spinning with their own distinct rhythm of
turmoil. There were no children here, but there was a childlike vulnerability in each face—a stark reminder that behind every facade lay
a story etched with heartbreak.

As I absorbed the scene, a gentle voice pierced the chaos. "You
don't belong in here," the orderly said. I turned to see a woman
whose age was betrayed only by the silver threads in her hair, her eyes
reflecting decades of empathy. "Why are you in here?" she asked.

I drew in a breath, exhaling the weight of my ordeal into words.
With each sentence, I unraveled the tapestry of my near demise,
revealing the struggle against my own shadow. She listened—not just
with her ears but with her soul—nodding at the right moments, her
presence a balm to my frayed spirit.

"Oh honey," she finally responded, her voice a soothing melody
amid discordant notes, "it sounds like you had a really bad day, but
you didn't do it. You didn't take your life and you went home. That
makes you just about as normal as everyone else and stronger than
most."

Her words were simple, yet they held the power of redemption.
"You had a moment of weakness and were able to get through it. You
should be out of here in no time, my friend." She offered a smile,
warm and genuine, then excused herself to attend to another patient
who had begun to spill coffee onto the linoleum floor, laughter bub-
bling from his lips.

Left alone with her assurance, I felt a flicker of hope stir within.
Her affirmation was a lifeline, pulling me back from the edge of self-
doubt. It was true—I had faced the abyss and chosen to walk away.
Perhaps that did not mark me as broken but as resilient.

In this place of fractured minds and spirits, I began to understand that our cracks are what allow us to connect with one another,
to empathize, to offer solace. We all have moments when darkness

whispers too convincingly, but it is our response to that call that defines us.

I stared out the window, where the world beyond seemed untouched by the turmoil within these walls. Yet in every person outside, there might be a hidden battle, a silent scream for help. The thought filled me with a sense of kinship that transcended the confines of "the Tower."

Life, with its unpredictable currents, had swept me into these depths, but it would soon release me back into the flow of the everyday. As I contemplated my return, I felt gratitude for the chance to begin anew, for the serendipity that had led me to safety.

Resilience, hope, luck—they were not just abstract concepts; they were tangible forces that had carried me through my darkest hour. Now, as I waited for release, I was ready to embrace them fully, ready to bet on the dawn after the longest night.

The fluorescent lights hummed above me, a monotonous drone that seemed to underline the sterile environment of the hospital's meeting room. A psychologist and a social worker sat across from me, their faces etched with professional concern. When they spoke, their words were both clinical and detached, as if discussing a case study rather than a man's life.

As the psychologist leaned back in her chair, pen poised over her notebook, she declared with a sense of finality, "You suffer from marijuana addiction syndrome." The words hung in the air like a heavy cloud, casting a shadow over our lengthy discussion about my recent ordeal. But this diagnosis felt like an absurd label, unable to capture the tangled web of circumstances that had led me to seek medical marijuana as my only relief. For years, it had been my lifeline, freeing me from the mind-numbing haze of morphine that had once consumed my every thought. It had helped me defeat a demon of my own making—a hopeless addiction to opiates, a result of the injury I sustained in the army. To reduce my struggle to such a simplistic cause that was actually a cure felt like a dismissal of the countless battles I had fought and won.

Yet I nodded, accepting their judgment with the same stoicism that had seen me through life's harshest storms. Three more days, they said, three days of observation and routine before I could step back into the world that had almost lost me.

I returned to my room, a small, impersonal space that somehow offered both solace and isolation. Time trickled by, measured out in scheduled meals, therapy sessions, and medication rounds. Shelly visited, her presence a balm to my weary spirit. She brought DVDs—old war movies we'd watched together, comedies that once made us laugh until tears streamed down our faces. We didn't speak much about the future or the past; we simply existed together, side by side, finding comfort in shared silence.

My mother came, too, her frail frame belying the strength within. She carried with her the scent of home, a whiff of the lilac bushes that bloomed beside the porch each spring. In her hands were more DVDs, a tangible connection to a life that continued beyond these walls. We watched them in the evenings, the flickering images a temporary escape from the reality of my surroundings.

As the days passed, I found a rhythm in the monotony, a strange peace in the knowing that each tick of the clock brought me closer to release. Reflection became my companion, a chance to peer inward and acknowledge the resilience that had kept me afloat. Hope sprouted like a delicate seedling in the fertile soil of my mind, nourished by the knowledge that luck—or perhaps fate—had spared me for a reason.

In moments of solitude, I contemplated the concept of luck. Was it truly just a random twist in the fabric of existence? Or was it something shaped by our own actions and desires? As I pondered this, I realized that my brush with the abyss had granted me a new perspective. Luck wasn't just about chance; it was about choices. The choice to keep fighting, to seek help, to embrace the potential for change.

As the third day dawned, I felt the weight of expectation settle upon my shoulders. Today, I would walk free. Free from the confines of "the Tower," free to face the complexities of a life interrupted but not ended. With each breath, I inhaled the promise of a fresh start, exhaling the doubts that lingered like shadows at the edge of my consciousness.

"Ready to go, Mr. Quayle?" an orderly asked, her smile warm and genuine.

"More ready than ever," I replied, my voice steady, my heart buoyant with the realization that this was not an end but a beginning. The chapter of despair was closing, and ahead lay a narrative yet unwritten, filled with the potential for redemption and growth.

"Let's get you checked out then," she said, leading me down the hall, my footsteps echoing with the sound of hope resounding off the sterile walls.

The doors opened, and I stepped into the crisp morning air, the sun's rays casting long shadows on the ground. It was the same world I had left behind, but I was not the same man. Transformed by adversity, tempered by experience, I was ready to weave the threads of resilience, hope, and luck into the tapestry of my life.

Stepping over the threshold of my home, the familiar scent of Shelly's cooking wafted through the air, a stark contrast to the sterile smell of "the Tower" that still lingered in my nostrils. The walls, once suffocating with memories of better days, now seemed to offer solace. I knew the path ahead was paved with difficult conversations, but the foundation beneath my feet felt solid, built on the resilience that had been my bedrock for so many tumultuous years.

Shelly stood at the kitchen counter, her back to me, chopping vegetables with a rhythm that spoke of routine and normalcy. It was a dance of domesticity that I had been absent from, moving to a tune I was uncertain I could still hear. The clink of her knife against the cutting board was a metronome to my racing heart as I prepared myself for the opening notes of our discourse.

"Welcome home," she said without turning around, her voice carrying a tremor that betrayed her composure as Mandy barked her greeting and licked my cheeks.

"Thank you," I replied, the words feeling like boulders tumbling from my lips. "We need to talk, I know."

"Let's eat first. You look like you could use a good meal," she suggested, her kindness wrapping around me like a warm blanket.

Dinner was a silent affair, punctuated by the clinking of cutlery and the unspoken thoughts that swirled around us like the steam rising from our plates. Each bite tasted of the future—uncertain yet filled with the nutrients necessary to sustain hope. We were two people, bound by vows and history, navigating the waters of forgiveness and understanding.

Afterward, we settled into the living room, the couch an island in the sea of our shared life. The conversation began tentatively, like the first few drops before a deluge. I spoke of the desolation that had driven me to the edge of existence, the darkness that nearly consumed me beneath the canopy of trees in the Metroparks. I told her about the moment of clarity, the divine intervention, Carrie Underwood's song that convinced me to drop the Glock into the mud and choose life.

She listened, her eyes never leaving mine, a mirror reflecting sorrow, relief, and love in equal measure. She held my hands in hers, small and strong, a lifeline cast across the chasm that had opened between us.

"Recovery won't happen overnight," I said, the weight of my words heavy with truth. "But I'm here, ready to face what comes. Together, we'll navigate this. I'm thankful for that."

A nod was her only response, her blonde hair catching the light, creating a halo effect that made me believe in angels on earth. Her faith in me was unwavering, even when mine had faltered.

In the days that followed, I sat with my mother, Elaine, her frail form a testament to the strength within. We didn't speak much, but our silence was a dialogue of its own, a conversation of souls that required no words. Deb, too, came with her own battles etched into the lines of her face. We shared a kinship of scars, each telling a story of survival against the odds.

Bernd brought laughter, a balm for the soul. His jokes, though sometimes ill-timed, reminded me that joy could be found even amid the rubble of despair. He was a beacon, guiding me back to the shores of camaraderie and fellowship.

Each interaction was a thread, weaving together the fabric of my existence. The tapestry was not without its frayed edges and dark patches, but it was mine—a portrait of a life lived fully, if not always wisely.

As the days turned into weeks, I found strength in the simple acts of living. A smile from Shelly, a kind word from Bernd, the warmth of my mother's hand in mine—all were reminders that I was luckier than most. Luck had been a companion of mine, often hiding in the shadows, waiting for the opportune moment to reveal itself.

I was Bobby Quayle, a man who had stared into the abyss and found the courage to step back. My journey was one of hope reborn from the ashes of despondency, a phoenix rising to meet the dawn of new possibilities. Each breath was a promise to myself and those who stood beside me—I would not waste this second chance.

There in the crucible of my own making, I forged a renewed sense of purpose. I was thankful, endlessly thankful, to be there, present and accountable, ready to dance once again to the song of life. It was not a cowardly retreat but a brave advance into the future, a melody composed of resilience, hope, and the ever-present serendipity that is luck.

CHAPTER 17

HITTING ROCK BOTTOM

I sat there, the weight of my world anchored to the creaky chair beneath me. Before me lay a sea of papers and figures, each one a reminder of choices made and roads taken. The store, once a bustling haven of commerce and community, stood silent now—a tomb to aspirations and dreams that had soared high but fallen hard in the wake of reality's harsh light.

"Bankruptcy seems like your best option," murmured my attorney, his voice barely disturbing the stillness of the room. He was a good man, seasoned by the law and life, yet even he looked uncomfortable delivering the verdict. "Which, at the end of the day, is no different than selling it and breaking even," added my accountant, her calculative eyes scanning columns of numbers that might as well have been ancient hieroglyphs for all the sense they made to me then. She wasn't wrong—Ricky-Bobby's slick promises had left me with nothing but debt and disillusionment.

As they spoke, I could only nod, feeling the strings of hope fraying within me. Yet I knew this was not an ending but a painful bend in the long road I tread. Bankruptcy was a word, a state, a moment in time—it would not define me. I had faced down challenges before, each one a forge in which my resolve was tempered.

The weeks passed, each day bleeding into the next, blurring lines between progress and stagnation. Then, when the skies of my life seemed their grayest, the phone rang—a familiar number but an unexpected voice pierced through the line. "I'm so sorry, Bobby, but I have to tell you that your father passed away this morning." The words fell from my stepmother's lips, heavy with grief that mirrored the sudden hollow in my chest. My hands trembled softly as the receiver slipped against my ear, the cold plastic an anchor to this new reality.

Her sobs merged with mine, two souls bound by a singular loss, strangers united in mourning. A man who had been more shadow than substance in my life had left this earth, taking with him the final embers of what might have been—an understanding, a reconciliation, now forever out of reach.

In that moment, amid the waves of sorrow, something within me shifted. I realized that each heartbreak was but a chapter, not the entire story. I was resilient, not because I was unbroken but because I allowed myself to feel every crack, every splinter, and chose to keep moving forward because, as Rocky says, that's how winning is done.

The quiet around me held a different texture now, tinged with both the sadness of endings and the quiet anticipation of beginnings. I wiped the tears from my cheeks, knowing that tomorrow beckoned with unseen opportunities, with the promise of renewal and the potential for joy yet undiscovered. "Life is an unyielding teacher," I whispered to the empty room, "and I am its tenacious student." With that, I stood up, ready to close the ledger on today and await the dawn of tomorrow.

As I stood before the assembly of somber faces, my own visage a mask of unanticipated grief, I came to a startling realization. The casket lay before me—my father's final resting place—and with it any chance of reconciliation lay buried in the ground. The sum total of our time together post-divorce might not have even filled a fortnight's worth of hours, yet here I was, heart fracturing beneath the weight of what would never be.

I grieved not just for the man who had been absent most of my life but for the potential of what could have been. The dreams of sitting down with him, looking him in the eye and releasing years of pent-up emotions, vanished with the echo of each clod of earth that struck his casket. He had left scars too deep on our family, wounds that perhaps even now were still raw upon my mother's tender heart.

"Goodbye, Dad," I whispered to the wind, my voice barely rising above a murmur. It was a farewell to both the man and the lingering hope of understanding and knowing him.

A few months drifted by, time's relentless march indifferent to human suffering, when Mandy's once vibrant eyes grew dull, and her lively steps became a disoriented wander through familiar rooms. She, who had been our joy, our constant companion through life's turbulence, now faced a journey we couldn't share.

The veterinarian's diagnosis was delivered with a compassionate gravity that only deepened the hollow pit in my stomach: a brain tumor. As she detailed the options, none offering a true reprieve, I felt Shelly's hand tighten around mine, her presence a silent pillar amid the crumbling ruins of our shared world.

We made the harrowing decision borne from love, yet it cleaved through us like a blade. In those final moments, as Mandy's gentle spirit slipped away, part of me went with her. Our home grew silent, a silence that seemed to absorb all light, all warmth.

Yet even in the depths of loss, I sought solace in carrying a piece of her with me. The gold cross resting against my chest bore the tangible remnants of a bond that stretched beyond the veil of mortality—a fusion of ashes and fur, an amulet of memories.

These twin sorrows—the death of my estranged father and the loss of my beloved pet—might have been enough to dim another's spirit. But within me, there stirred a quiet defiance, an ember of hope refusing to be extinguished. My resilience, tested time and again, did not falter; it was the steel upon which my character was forged.

Day bled into night, and night into day, each cycle a reminder that life's narrative is composed of both joy and pain, interwoven in a tapestry of experience. And with each sunrise, I reminded myself that the story was not over. There was more to be written, more to be lived. "Out of these ashes will rise a new chapter," I assured my reflection in the mirror. With each step forward, I carried the legacy of lost loved ones and the certainty that their lessons would guide me toward a future ripe with possibility.

The silence in the house was like a vacuum, pulling at the fringes of my reality. I stood there, in the doorway, key still dangling from the lock, struck by the stark emptiness that greeted me. My gaze traced the outlines where furniture once anchored our lives together, now just dusty impressions on the carpet—a testament to what had been and what was no more.

Shelly's disdain for bankruptcy had always been palpable, woven tightly into her moral fabric. But life, as I've learned, rarely adheres to the black-and-white principles we clutch so dearly. Our attorney's voice still echoed, his words attempting to dismantle the stigma she felt: "Bankruptcy can be a responsible choice, a tool for a fresh start." And the accountant, with his pragmatic tone, pointing out that even financial titans had fallen only to rise anew. It took time, but eventually, Shelly nodded, her agreement coming as a surrender rather than acceptance.

Our marriage, already weathering storms of difference and disparity, found itself adrift in a sea of loss and looming failure. The chasm between us grew with each trial, the echoes of our love lost in the void. We were a study in contrasts; she was the still water to my relentless wave, the quiet night to my raging storm. Yet it was not our differences that undid us but the shared burdens that became unbearable.

The once fruitless sessions of counseling had transformed into a rigid, repetitive dance of going through the motions without making any real progress. The writing on the wall was clear—we were simply postponing the inevitable. And then, on that fateful day, as I struggled to adjust to my new job and all its accompanying responsibilities, Shelly made a decisive move.

Our mutual love for Mandy, once the unbreakable bond between us, no longer held any weight to keep our relationship intact due to her passing. She packed up her entire life, including our other beloved dog Wags, leaving behind only the remnants of our shattered existence. The emptiness left in their absence felt like a gaping wound, serving as a constant reminder of all that I had lost. As I looked around at the desolate space that was once our shared home, it was impossible to ignore the harsh reality of our broken relationship.

But amid the hollow echo of an emptied home, I found a certain liberty—a freedom to redefine myself without the expectations or judgments of another. There was resilience within me yet, a stubborn flame that would not be snuffed out by the gusts of misfortune. My heart may have ached for Wags' cheerful bark and the soft warmth she brought to our lives, but I understood this was part of a larger narrative, one where change was both the protagonist and the antagonist.

I picked up the gold cross that hung around my neck, thumb grazing over the textured surface that held Mandy's essence, her memory a mingling of sorrow and solace. It was a talisman of continuity, a link to the love that endured beyond physical presence. And in that moment of introspection, I realized that while some chapters had ended, my story was far from over.

"Tomorrow," I whispered to the empty room, "is ripe with unknowns and unturned stones." My voice was steady, my resolve firmer than it had been in months. Closing the door behind me, I left the past where it belonged and turned my face toward the dawning future, ready to embrace whatever came next with hope cradled in one hand and determination in the other.

The cool touch of the hardwood floor beneath me was a stark contrast to the warmth of the memories that swirled around the hollow expanse of our living room. "Life ain't all sunshine and rainbows, it's a very mean and nasty place, and it will beat you into the ground if you let it." The words of Rocky Balboa, always more poet than pugilist to me, reverberated in my mind as I sat there, surrounded by echoes of laughter and tears once shared with Shelly.

Twenty years of life together, our journey had been like a meandering river, now departed from its familiar banks. We'd charted our course through calm waters and storms, only to find ourselves adrift, navigating the currents separately. In Texas, we'd sought refuge from one tempest, only to return and face another.

A wry smile crossed my lips as I recalled Mandy, our dog with the spirit of a comet, who once blazed through this very room. Her legs had churned with such joyous abandon that day that she seemed to believe she could outrun the wind itself. And then—bang! Into the glass patio doors she crashed, her surprise at the sudden barrier almost comical. I remember how she just sat there afterward, a puzzled look softening her energetic eyes as if questioning the existence of unseen walls. Could such an impact have planted the seeds of her later illness? The thought was a splinter in my heart.

Yet as I mourned her loss, along with the absence of my father and the void left by Shelly, I recognized within the silence a presence that had been masked by the cacophony of everyday life—a resilience, quiet but unyielding. It was not the end of my story but a challenging chapter that demanded to be lived and overcome.

In the stillness, I found solace in the simplicity of being. The weight of the past, though heavy, was a testament to strength, not burden. My father, whom I never truly knew, left a legacy of lessons learned in his absence. Mandy, with her boundless energy and innocence, taught me to embrace the present, even when it collided with the unexpected. And Shelly…she had shared a dance with me in the sun and shadows, each step a part of a greater whole.

Time had become a relentless tide, washing over me as I remained anchored on the hardwood floor, awash in the silence of my hollowed home. The walls seemed to absorb the echo of Mandy's playful barks, her bright eyes and wagging tail painting a vivid picture in the canvas of my mind. I closed my eyes, and for a moment, I could feel the softness of her fur beneath my hands, her comforting presence a balm to the loneliness that clung to me like a second skin.

I sighed, the sound lonely in the emptiness. Shelly's laughter used to ring out here, our differences once the sparks that lit fires of passion and frustration alike. Now all that remained was the residue of memories, the bitter mingling with the sweet. Our love had been a tempest, beautiful and destructive. I had known even then, with each storm weathered, that our paths were diverging, our rhythms too discordant to maintain the dance we had begun in our youth.

Shelly had always been ahead of the curve, her intuition unnervingly precise, and so it was no surprise she had taken the first step away. I couldn't blame her; freedom beckoned us both to new horizons. Despite the hollow ache of her absence, I harbored no ill will.

"May you find peace," I murmured into the void, an earnest wish for her future.

The clock's hands crept forward, indifferent to my reverie, urging me to rise. A deep weariness settled in my bones, yet there was a spark—a flicker of something undeniably alive within me. With effort, I stood, legs stiff from hours spent motionless, and made my way through the ghostly remnants of my former life.

As the dusk crept in, casting long shadows across the empty room, I felt the flicker of hope ignite within me. Tomorrow beckoned with its myriad possibilities, an unwritten page in the book of my life. Grief would not consume me; I would not allow it to. Instead, I would carry forward the love and lessons of those I cherished, crafting from their memory a mosaic of hope and determination.

Ascending the stairs felt akin to climbing a mountain—each step a testament to the trials I had endured, to the resilience etched into the very marrow of my being. The bedroom door creaked open, revealing the moonlight spilling through the window, casting long shadows that stretched across the bare floor.

As I laid down, the bed felt foreign without the familiar weight of another beside me, without the soft snoring of a loyal canine companion. But within the stillness, I found solace. Tomorrow held no promises, but it was ripe with possibility. The slate was clean, the past a collection of lessons learned, and the future a field waiting to be sown with new dreams.

"Tomorrow," I whispered to the night, a simple word heavy with potential. My eyelids grew heavy, and as I drifted into sleep, I clung to the hope that dawn would bring with it the promise of reinvention, a chance to forge a path defined by wisdom gained through hardship and the courage to embrace the unknown.

The end of one chapter marked the beginning of another, and I was the author of my own story—bruised but unbroken, ready to pen the next lines with a heart open to whatever twists of fate awaited.

CHAPTER 18

A New Path Forward

The morning light seeped in through the half-open blinds, casting a muted glow across the bedroom. My eyes flickered open, and for a brief moment, I lay still in the silence that was heavier than the usual cacophony of sounds. There was no clinking of coffee mugs, no swish of fabric as Shelly prepared for work, no eager barks from Wags demanding her playtime. It took my groggy mind a moment to catch up with reality, one where these sounds wouldn't greet me again.

I sat up, rubbing the sleep from my eyes, and let out a deep breath. As the emptiness of the room enveloped me, memories of the previous night crept back. The house was just an echo chamber now; Shelly's absence had turned it so. She was gone, her departure marking the end of an era in my life. A pang of sorrow tugged at my heart, but deeper within, acceptance settled like sediment at the bottom of a once-turbulent river. It was for the best—for both of us.

Dragging myself out of bed, I shuffled into the kitchen and mechanically scooped coffee grounds into the maker. The rich aroma soon filled the small space, a comforting ritual in an unmoored world. With a steaming mug in hand, I sank into the worn fabric of the couch and clicked on the morning news. The anchors' voices were a familiar backdrop as I let my mind wander, retracing the contours of two decades within these walls.

A lot of life was lived here—good times, tough times—they all mingled together in a tapestry of experience. The thought brought Mandy to the forefront of my memories, our beloved Border Collie mix who had long since passed but remained a beacon of joy in my recollections. The ghost of a smile graced my lips as I pictured her "Woo-woos," that unique sound, halfway between a howl and bark, her way of expressing pure happiness or urging me to join in her play. Her antics with Wags, their morning frolics in the yard, it was as if they were imploring me to seize the day with the same fervor.

And I would, I resolved silently. Maybe not with the same carefree abandon as Mandy, but with determination. Life had knocked me down more times than I cared to count, but it had also taught me the value of standing back up. This quiet morning marked the beginning of another chapter, one where resilience was my guiding force and hope my constant companion.

The past twenty years were etched into the fabric of this house, a testament to both triumphs and trials. But as I sipped my coffee, letting its warmth spread through me, the weight of history felt lighter. There was a future to be written, and I was the author of my own destiny. With every sip, the shadows of doubt receded, replaced by the light of possibility.

The mattress store was quiet that morning, the kind of hush that seems to amplify every minor sound. The fluorescent lights hummed overhead as I straightened out a row of pillows on one of the display beds, my movements mechanical. The new job—it was supposed to be a stopgap, something to tide me over. But as I stood there in my drab uniform, surrounded by mattresses that promised dreams they couldn't deliver, it felt like a mockery of my abilities.

"Remember, Bobby, 'Our comfort guarantees are unparalleled,'" the manager, Jimmy, recited with an eagerness that grated on my nerves. He was a good kid, barely into his twenties, but right then, he felt like another symbol of my misdirection. "Customers need to feel they're making the best choice for their sleep health."

"Sleep health," I muttered under my breath. After decades of serving my country, analyzing intelligence, I found myself peddling sleep rather than safeguarding security. And the script—the endless, soulless script—seemed like chains binding me to mediocrity.

My patience was a thinning wire, and Jimmy's insistent coaching snipped it clean through. Handing him my nametag, I met his confused gaze with a level stare. "I wish you luck, son," I said, my voice steady despite the churn of uncertainty within me. "But this isn't where I'm meant to end up."

He tried to protest, but I left without looking back. The decision was impulsive, maybe even foolish, yet as I walked out into the crisp air of freedom, my spirit soared. There was something liberating about choosing potential hardship over comfortable despair.

As weeks turned into months, the house became less a home and more a reminder of all that had transpired within its walls. Shelly's absence had hollowed it out, leaving behind only the echo of old memories. Deciding to sell was logical; the sprawling space was unnecessary for one, and the financial strain of the mortgage was a weight I could do without.

The housing market was still reeling, trying to find its footing after the collapse years ago. My realtor, a man with a practiced smile and optimistic clichés, assured me we'd find a buyer. And he did, but for a price that should have been much higher. The sale wasn't lucrative, but it was enough—a clean break, financially and emotionally.

Sitting at the dining room table now cluttered with boxes rather than family meals, I signed the papers with a mix of reluctance and relief. In the margin, where the ink bled just slightly onto the grainy paper, I scrawled a small note: "To new beginnings."

The house would soon belong to strangers, who'd fill it with their own laughter and tears. But as I looked around one last time, I realized that change was not synonymous with loss. It was merely the turning of a page, a chance to author a new chapter in a life that was still mine to command.

In those final moments, as the sun dipped low, casting long shadows across the yard I had tended with love and sweat, I felt the contours of hope solidifying within me. Yes, there were uncertainties ahead, battles to be fought, dreams to chase. But the resilience that had carried me through darker times pulsed within, a silent promise that whatever lay ahead, I was ready.

And so with the chapter of this house coming to a close, I stepped into the unknown with a heart open to whatever fortune had in store. Because while fate had dealt me a difficult hand, it was my tenacity, my unyielding hope, that would shape the days to come.

The fire crackled, breaking the silence of the evening as I watched the flames lick the sky, their warm glow a stark contrast to the coolness settling in my bones. This was it—the last night in the home that had been a witness to the tapestry of my life for twenty long years. Sitting alone on the wooden bench that still held the scent of sawdust from my own hands, I felt the weight of memories pressing down upon me.

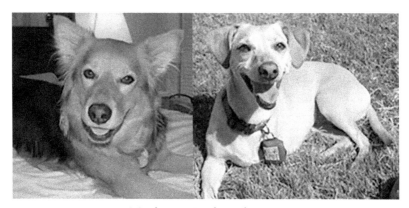

My dogs, Mandy and Wags.

In the dance of shadows cast by the firelight, I could almost make out Mandy's joyful form bounding across the yard, her spirit as alive as ever in my heart. She would have loved this fire, the excitement of the flickering light and the chance to be close, always so eager for companionship and play. The memory of her intelligence brought a sad smile to my lips; she had been more than just a pet— she was a friend and a family member, one whose absence left a void no amount of time seemed capable of filling.

I remembered our routine with such clarity it hurt: the way she'd anticipate my every turn as I mowed the lawn, dropping her ball into my path, trusting I'd send it flying for her to chase. It was a simple joy, but in its simplicity lay the beauty of life we often overlook. All at once, I missed those days fiercely, the uncomplicated happiness of shared moments.

As tears found their way down weathered cheeks, unchecked and unashamed, they were not just for Mandy or the past but for the acknowledgment of change, of letting go. Yet within that sorrow, there sparked a flame of something else—hope, perhaps, or the beginning of acceptance. My life had been a rugged terrain, each hill and valley shaping the man I had become. And here I was, preparing to leave behind the familiar, the comfortable—even if it was tinged with pain.

The fire's warmth seeped into my skin, a gentle reminder that life was still coursing through these aging veins. I had stood against storms before, had learned to bend when necessary, and to stand tall when it mattered most. As the blaze before me consumed the remnants of some forgotten tree, it whispered a promise of renewal, of life continuing in cycles of growth and decay.

"New beginnings," I murmured into the night air, the words a balm to the sting of parting. With every crackle and pop from the fire pit, I let fragments of the past drift away, making room for what was yet to come. There would be new lawns to mow, new friends to meet, perhaps even new dogs to chase after thrown balls.

The house would soon echo with the laughter and footsteps of another family, and that was how it should be. Like the coals turning to ash in the pit, I recognized the necessity of moving on, of transformation. I had my share of scars, sure, but they were medals of survival, proof I could weather whatever lay ahead.

The fire crackled, a soft symphony to accompany the theater of memories playing out in my mind. I stood up from the bench, stretching legs that felt as weathered as the wooden planks beneath me. Stepping off the patio, I wandered into the yard, my hands brushing against the dew-kissed leaves that bordered the garden.

Each touch was a goodbye, a silent thank you to the earth that had flourished under my care.

I remembered the laughter that had once filled this space, the clinking of glasses, and the murmur of conversations spilling out like music from an unseen radio. We had hosted countless family gatherings here, birthdays where candles flickered as wishes were whispered, anniversaries where old stories were polished and presented anew. The aroma of grilled meats and homemade pies had mingled with the scent of jasmine and lilac, creating a perfume unique to this place, to these moments.

I paused before the rosebushes, their blooms a testament to patience and persistence. It wasn't just plants I had nurtured here but relationships too. This green haven bore witness to reconciliations and partings, to quiet confessions and raucous declarations. I smiled at the thought of the next family continuing the tradition, their own milestones rooted amid the foliage.

With each step through the yard, the years unfolded around me, a tapestry woven from threads of joy and sorrow. This house, this land, they held echoes of Shelly's laughter, hints of her presence in every corner. And though we had parted, what we shared remained embedded in the very foundations of this home. My fingers traced the etched letters of our surname in the concrete path—our indelible mark on a place that had cradled two decades of our lives.

As dawn approached, a lightness settled within me. The weight of the past, while always a part of me, no longer anchored me to this spot. I gazed upon my horticultural masterpiece one last time, acknowledging the labor of love it represented. From the soil, I had coaxed forth life, beauty, and sanctuary, much like the resilience I mustered to rebuild my own life, time and again.

"Thank you," I whispered to the garden, to the house, to the ghosts of days gone by. "For everything." My voice was steady, a calm certainty flowing through the words. It was an ending, yes, but also a beginning. Each memory, whether dipped in happiness or shaded with regret, was a steppingstone leading me to tomorrow.

Turning back toward the fire, I knew the embers of my history here would continue to glow long after I had gone. They were not chains but rather beacons, illuminating the strength I had found in adversity, the hope that sprouted from despair. I was ready to plant new dreams in fresh soil, to cultivate a future lined with possibility.

With the fire dwindling, I rose from the bench, casting one last glance at the place that had been my haven. Tomorrow, I would step into the unknown, carrying with me the resilience that had seen me through darker times. I was ready to turn the page, to embrace the unwritten story of my life with an open heart.

"Here's to fresh starts," I said to the stars peeking through the darkening sky. They twinkled back, like silent witnesses to my quiet resolve. With each step I took away from the fire, from the house, from all that had been, I felt lighter, as though shedding a skin that no longer fit. It was time to move forward, to see what fortune had in store for a man who refused to give up.

And as the embers faded, so did the grip of the past, leaving behind the soft glow of anticipation for a dawn yet to break.

"Forward," I said to myself, the promise of the rising sun painting the horizon with hues of change. "Always forward." The silhouette of the house receded as I walked away, its outline a part of me yet distinct, like the closing chapter of a well-loved book, its lessons etched deep in my soul.

The first glimmer of dawn peeked through the blinds as I lugged the last of my boxes down the familiar creaking steps. The U-Haul truck sat like a hulking yellow beast in the driveway, yawning open to swallow the remnants of a life once shared. The son of my neighbor, a strapping young lad with more brawn than years, hoisted my weathered couch with an ease that made my own muscles twinge in envy.

"Almost there, Mr. Quayle," he said cheerily, his breath visible in the crisp morning air. His friends, a motley crew of energetic youths, buzzed around the property, a whirlwind of activity and laughter, a stark contrast to the stillness that had settled over the house.

As they worked, I found myself in the now-bare living room, my fingers tracing the groove where a picture frame used to hang—a photo that captured a moment when smiles were easy and the future seemed a vast, unexplored territory. With each empty shelf and silent corner, the echo of what was grew fainter, and in its place, a quiet determination began to hum.

It was amid the dust motes and the scent of lemon cleaner that inspiration struck—a sudden, brilliant flash. The GI Bill, a resource earned but untouched, a path not taken that now beckoned me toward a horizon I hadn't dared to contemplate in years. The idea unfurled within me, a seedling pushing through the cracks of hardened soil.

The following day, I stood outside the university's veteran services office, the emblem of my military past polished and gleaming on the door. My heart hammered a staccato rhythm against my ribs—was I ready for this? Was it too late to reinvent oneself, to step back into the classroom where youth would be my fellow companions?

"Never too late," I muttered under my breath, a mantra to bolster the certainty that wavered. My hand pushed open the door, and I was greeted by the sight of a wall adorned with flags and photographs, each one telling stories of service and sacrifice.

"Can I help you?" a voice, warm and welcoming, cut through my reverie.

"Yes," I replied, feeling the weight of my years and experiences as assets rather than burdens. "I'm here to talk about enrolling under the GI Bill."

The representative—competent, also a veteran, understanding eyes meeting mine—nodded and gestured to a seat across from his desk. As he outlined forms and schedules, the reality of my decision took shape, molding itself into a tangible plan.

"Classes start in a couple of weeks, so we'll need to get you registered quickly," he explained, his efficiency a lifeline thrown across the chasm of uncertainty.

"Thank you," I said, the gratitude genuine and deep. It wasn't just for his guidance but for the universe conspiring to present this opportunity when I most needed direction.

With registration papers clutched in my hand, a symbol of commitment and a passport to a new beginning, I left the campus with my head held high. The apartment complex that awaited me was no longer a retreat but a launchpad, a base camp for the ascent to come.

"Forward," I whispered again, a promise to myself, to Mandy's memory, and to the echoes of laughter that lingered in the home I'd left behind. This time, the word carried more than hope—it was imbued with action, with the next step already in motion beneath my feet. Forward into learning, growth, and the uncharted terrain of a world that was, remarkably, still full of possibility.

The first thing I noticed in my new apartment was the echo. Each footstep, each creak of an empty cupboard, resonated with the starkness of a blank canvas. But it was more than emptiness; it was potential. I spent those initial days before classes started working on my apartment. I turned my attention to furnishing the place. The act of selecting a couch, a bed, and a dining table felt almost ceremonial, as though each piece I brought into this space was a declaration: this was my new life. I chose a deep blue for the sofa, thinking how it mirrored the steadfastness I sought within myself. As I unpacked pots and pans, the clatter seemed less like noise and more like the percussion of progress.

A television found its place against the wall, not so much for the background noise it provided but as a reminder that the world outside continued to spin, and I was still a part of it. Kitchenware and utensils filled drawers that Shelly had left hollow. Standing back, hands on my hips, I surveyed my work: a home reforged from the remnants of an old one. Then time accelerated, as it has a habit of doing when life begins anew. Nearly a year whisked by before I could catch my breath.

The campus grounds became familiar territory, trodden by feet that grew surer with each passing day. I had become one of the "non-traditional students," a polite term for the gray at my temples and the lines etched around my eyes—marks of experience rather than age, I told myself.

Late one night, after classes, I clicked on the illuminated screen, my index finger hesitating just a fraction of a second before sending my status into the ether. The glow from the computer barely lit up the dimly lit room, where the shadows seemed to echo my solitary state. It had been decades since I had dipped my toes into the murky waters of the dating pool, and frankly, the temperature hadn't become any more inviting with time.

"Trying to find someone genuine at this age is like searching for a needle in a stack of needles," I typed, a wry smile touching my lips as I considered the metaphor. It was a risky move—airing my frustrations so publicly—but there was a cathartic release in just putting it out there. I hit "Post" and leaned back in my chair, a soft sigh escaping me. Dating in your late forties and fifties, I mused, wasn't just challenging; it was an exercise in patience and, often, in futility.

Most evenings were spent sifting through profiles that read more like car advertisements than glimpses into someone's soul. It felt as if all the good ones were indeed taken, leaving behind a landscape littered with the remnants of relationships past, each person carrying their own set of luggage heavy enough to fill a cargo hold.

But then something unexpected happened. A notification pinged, and there she was—Cheryl, the girl who had starred in my high school dreams, her name now highlighted in blue on my screen. We had been friends on Facebook, connected by our shared history, though we had never really conversed beyond the occasional "like" or generic holiday greeting. She hadn't changed much—the same bright, beautiful blue eyes that used to catch the sunlight in the school corridors now peered out from her profile picture, her smile just as infectious as I remembered. In that moment, nostalgia washed over me, a wave of memories flooding back with the force of a riptide.

"It's probably because you're too nice, Bobby, that's why you're struggling to meet someone," she had commented on my post, a simple acknowledgment that felt like a lifeline thrown across the digital divide. And suddenly, the prospect of finding companionship didn't seem quite so bleak. The idea of Cheryl, with her easy laugh and the way she used to tuck her hair behind her ear when she was deep in thought, filled the room with a warmth that had been absent for far too long. It was a small step, that single comment, but it spurred a hope within me that had lain dormant beneath layers of cynicism and disappointment. Maybe, just maybe, the universe had a funny way of circling back, of offering second chances when you least expect them. First, I clicked on her profile... "Single" it read beneath her relationship status.

"What?" I said aloud as I looked at her profile in disbelief. As I prepared to type a response, I allowed myself to believe in the possibility of new beginnings, my heart quietly whispering that not all was lost to time.

"Looks like we're in the same boat," I replied, the cursor blinking in rhythm with the tentative beat of my heart. "Care to navigate these waters together?" It was an invitation, a hand extended across years and pixels, a shot at rediscovering a connection that might have been written in the stars all those years ago. And as I waited for her reply, I realized that no matter how vast the sea of uncertainty, one thing remained true—I was a sailor who had weathered many storms, and I was ready to set sail once again.

Staring at the screen, I watched as the chat notification blinked with an energy that seemed to mock my hesitation. It had been a simple online jest about the trials of dating past one's prime, but Cheryl's reply cut through the digital noise with the unexpected sharpness of truth. "It's probably because you're too nice, Bobby!" The words seemed to leap off the page.

With a mixture of curiosity and old longing, I navigated to her profile. There it was, "Single"—a status that struck me as both a beacon of possibility and a puzzle. Cheryl, with her gentle laugh that echoed through high school hallways and the kindness in her eyes that made even the most mundane days sparkle was unspoken for? Time had etched experience into us both, yet here she was, the girl who once filled my teenage days with silent yearning, now a woman of grace on my computer screen.

CHAPTER 19

ROMANCE BLOSSOMS AND ANOTHER UNIQUE OPPORTUNITY

The weeks that followed were a blur of messages and late-night conversations. Each keystroke, each shared memory, felt like a step closer to something remarkable. The day I finally mustered the courage to ask for her number, my voice wavered with a vulnerability I hadn't known since those youthful days of uncertainty. When we started dating, the connection was instantaneous, as if all the scattered pieces of my past were aligning to form a picture I had never before seen so clearly.

As Cheryl and I began to bond and become better acquainted, a unique opportunity emerged from being a student. It was the highly coveted internship required by my university, a crucial part of the college experience that I chose to participate in despite having enough experience to potentially waive it.

To my luck, the Republican National Convention was taking place in Cleveland that year, with all eyes on the upcoming presidential election. To my delight, I was selected to intern for an esteemed international news network at the RNC. My heart raced with excitement as I anticipated being a part of such a historic event, regardless of my political views.

My role was to escort important guests to and from the green room and assist the news personalities whenever needed. Through this job, I had the chance to meet countless famous celebrities and influential political figures, leaving me both starstruck and dizzy. The only tangible evidence of this incredible experience were the selfies I managed to snap along the way.

Life became a whirlwind of textbooks and tender moments. As I poured over my studies, Cheryl became both my sanctuary and muse, inspiring me to push through every challenge with her unwavering support. We found ourselves wrapped up in the kind of love that I had almost convinced myself didn't exist—at least not for me, not after everything.

Eighteen months vanished like mist in the morning sun. I found a rhythm in the routine of exams and evenings spent with Cheryl, each day building upon the last, constructing a future bright with promise. Yet sometimes when the night grew still and the world outside my window faded into shadows, a chill would grip my heart. The memory of a cold day in Metroparks, where despair had nearly won, crept into my thoughts. The metallic taste of desperation lingered, a stark reminder of what could have been.

Classes were a mosaic of fresh faces, young enough to be my children, and professors who sometimes paused when they caught my gaze, perhaps recognizing a peer rather than a pupil. It was a reminder of the diversity of life's paths, and I took comfort in knowing that learning was not confined to the youthful.

In lecture halls, I listened intently, absorbing knowledge like a sponge that had been dry for too long. I scribbled notes, engaged in discussions, and found that my life experiences often provided a unique perspective that enriched classroom debates. I wasn't just a student; I was a contributor.

There were moments between the turning of pages and the scratching of pens, where I allowed myself to look inward. I thought of Mandy's joyous bark, the firepit's last dance and Shelly's absence now a distant shadow. And there, amid textbooks and term papers, I embraced a truth: my story was still being written.

"Perseverance" became my silent mantra. With each chapter read and each assignment completed, it whispered encouragement, promising that past failures were merely stepping stones to future triumphs. And as I walked through the campus—a man nearing fifty surrounded by youth—I realized that I wasn't just moving forward; I was ascending.

To the outside observer, I might have appeared a solitary figure among a sea of exuberance. Yet within, I was anything but alone. I carried the strength of those I had loved, the lessons from every tumble, and the resilience that had become as much a part of me as the air I breathed. My journey was solitary, yes, but it was also universal—the unyielding march of the human spirit, ever hopeful, ever striving.

And so amid the bustle of campus life, the flicker of new beginnings colored my world with shades of optimism. I had weathered storms, navigated loss, and emerged not unscathed but undefeated. A testament, perhaps, to the extraordinary power of ordinary courage.

Turning the page of my hefty textbook, I felt an energy that was both alien and exhilarating—a vitality that had nothing to do with my age. I let out a quiet chuckle, thinking how I must look to these young college students, with my lined face and determined eyes among their youthful exuberance. Yet as the professor spoke about economic theories, I realized that my life's tapestry was rich with experience that could weave into these lessons something real and tangible.

I found myself raising my hand, contributing insights from years in the field that textbooks couldn't encapsulate. And they listened—these kids who were the age of my own children might have been, if I had them. Their eager faces turned toward me, some with curiosity, others with respect that was hard-earned. In those moments, knowledge flowed both ways, and I savored the exchange like a rare commodity.

My assignments were more than tasks; they were challenges that I relished conquering. Every A marked on my papers was a silent nod to the resilience that had carried me through darker times. The extra credit wasn't for padding a grade—it was proof to myself that I could still exceed expectations, my own most of all.

As I walked across the stage to receive my diploma, business administration with a minor in criminal justice inscribed upon it, I couldn't help but feel a sense of surrealism. This was the culmination of years of hard work and determination, a testament to the strength and resilience that had carried me through so many challenges.

Magna cum laude—some may have called it an honor, but to me, it was the physical manifestation of sheer willpower. As I shook hands with professors and peers alike, the weight of the parchment seemed to carry all the gravity of my former life's trials and triumphs.

My mother and sister sat in the audience, their eyes shining with pride as they watched me walk across that stage. My sister's husband, Robert, had also come to support me, and my new wife, Cheryl, was by my side as well. It was a bittersweet moment—my father wasn't there to witness this achievement, but I knew he would have been proud.

"Congratulations, Mr. Quayle," said the Dean, his handshake firm and meaningful. "Your dedication is inspiring."

"Thank you," I replied with genuine humility, "but it's never too late to add another chapter to your story."

I had woven my past—a patchwork of intelligence analysis and banking—into this new academic achievement. It felt fitting then that I also emerged from my collegiate rebirth with a certification in anti-money laundering. A once nebulous career path now lay before me, clear and inviting: financial crimes investigations beckoned, and I stepped toward it with newfound purpose.

Walking out of the auditorium, diploma in hand, a fresh sense of hope unfurled within me. Like a seedling pushing through soil after a harsh winter, I was proof that growth is not only the domain of the young or the unscathed. The campus behind me was awash with students celebrating, their laughter and chatter a vibrant backdrop to my introspective victory.

As I moved forward, my mind danced between thoughts of Mandy's playful bark and the crisp edges of my future business cards, embossed with titles yet to be claimed. My story, written with grit and grace, was still unfolding. And with each step, I embraced the great unknown, armed with an education earned not just in lecture halls, but in the theater of life itself.

I couldn't help but remember that fateful day in the Metroparks. I shook the memory away, just as I brushed the autumn leaves off my jacket after a long walk. But as I did, I felt a sense of thankfulness well up within my soul. The choice I made not to pull the trigger had set me on a new path, one of redemption and rebirth guided by a higher power.

Each morning as I faced myself in the mirror, I saw someone stronger, someone who had walked through many fires and emerged each time with an unbreakable spirit. For it was not luck or chance that brought me to this point but the grace of God and his divine hand in my life. He had taken control and steered me in a new direction, one filled with hope and purpose.

And as I stepped out into each new day, I carried with me the understanding that second chances were not just mere coincidences but precious gifts from above. And I was determined to honor mine every single day, grateful for every breath and every step forward.

Like Carrie sang about in her song, Jesus truly took the wheel in my life. He has guided me through trials and challenges, molding me into a better person filled with love, faith, and gratitude. As I reflect on my journey thus far, I am humbled and blessed to have made it this far with him by my side.

As we celebrated afterward with dinner at a lavish, upscale restaurant, surrounded by the warm embrace of loved ones and the tantalizing aroma of decadent food, I couldn't help but reflect on the incredible journey that had brought me to this moment. From my humble beginnings as a poor, abused child, lost and searching for meaning in life, to my valiant service in the army and eventual return home, battling through tumultuous relationships and financial hardships, to enduring the heart-wrenching loss of cherished family members—the fact that I now stand tall as a successful graduate with boundless opportunities ahead is nothing short of miraculous. Every obstacle overcome, every scar earned, has only made this triumph all the sweeter.

Amid laughter and congratulations from family and friends, Cheryl leaned over and whispered in my ear, "I am so proud of you."

And for once in my life, I believed those words without any hint of doubt or hesitation.

This day marked not only an academic accomplishment for me but also a personal victory—a shedding of old doubts and insecurities. As we raised our glasses for a toast that evening, I knew that this was just the beginning. The world was wide open now, full of possibilities waiting for me to explore and conquer.

With the support of my loved ones, I was ready.

CHAPTER 20

REFLECTION AND GROWTH

I stand at the summit of a small hill in the Metroparks where Cheryl and I often come to clear our heads, the city of Berea sprawled out below us like a vast, breathing entity. The air is crisp, and the scent of fresh grass fills my lungs as I look across the horizon, contemplating the winding road that has led me here. It's been a journey marked by both grace and grit, an odyssey of highs and lows that could fill volumes.

As I gaze upon the setting sun, its dying light casting a golden glow over the world, I can't help but feel a sense of awe for the sheer tenacity of the human spirit. Mine is not a tale spun from grandeur or fame but rather one stitched together with the threads of perseverance and faith. I'm no hero; just Bobby Quayle, a guy who's managed to keep on keeping on, even when the chips were down.

You see, life has thrown its fair share of punches my way. Some knocked the wind right out of me, left me gasping for air on the canvas, wondering if I'd ever rise again. But it's in those moments, the ones where hope seems nothing more than a distant flicker, that something extraordinary happens. You find strength that you never knew you had. You push back against the despair, plant your feet, and stand tall once more.

It's in this quiet reflection that I realize the power of sharing one's story. There's someone out there, maybe sitting on their own hilltop or nursing a cup of coffee in a crowded cafe, who needs to hear that they're not alone. That their battles aren't fought in solitude and that victory, though elusive, is worth the scars.

So I pen these words, not as a boast or a lecture but as an open hand extended in solidarity. To that person, you might be feeling beaten and broken, but I've been there too. And I promise you, the darkness doesn't last forever. No pit is so deep that light cannot reach it. And that light, sometimes it comes from places unexpected or from within yourself.

If my life has taught me anything, it's that resilience isn't just the ability to endure; it's the courage to continue moving forward, one uncertain step at a time. Every challenge faced, every obstacle overcome, it's all part of a grander design, a tapestry woven with threads of trials and triumphs.

The sun dips below the horizon now, leaving a symphony of purple and orange streaks in its wake. The beauty of it, ephemeral yet eternal, mirrors the very essence of our struggles. They shape us, mold us into beings of substance, character etched into our very souls.

"Let's head back," Cheryl says, her hand finding mine, warm and reassuring. Her faith in me has been an unyielding pillar, a testament to the power of love through life's tempests.

"Sure thing," I reply, squeezing her hand gently.

We descend the hill together, side by side, the weight of the past a little lighter with each step. The future, unknown as it may be, holds no terror for me. For in my heart, I carry the unwavering belief that no matter how daunting the path ahead, there is always light at the end of the tunnel. And with faith as my compass, I will navigate whatever comes next, thriving against the odds.

*****

As I sit quietly on the wooden bench in the Metroparks that's become a sanctuary for my thoughts, I watch the people passing by. Each one carries their own invisible burdens, their faces etched with the stories of their lives. There's an old man feeding pigeons, his hands trembling slightly with age or emotion—I can't tell which. A young woman sits alone, headphones in, her eyes distant as if searching for answers in the lyrics of a song only she can hear.

I've come to understand that life doesn't discriminate when it delivers hardship; it's an impartial teacher of tough lessons. And it's in these quiet moments of reflection that I am reminded above all else to be good to those around me. We're all participants in the same unpredictable journey, and none of us is privy to the entirety of another's story—their battles fought in silence, their private defeats and victories.

Gazing at the scene before me, a sense of kinship fills my chest. These strangers are unknowingly part of my narrative, just as I am a footnote in theirs. It's incumbent upon us to offer kindness to forgive the faults and failings we so readily see in ourselves and others. For we're bound by a common desire: to be accepted and loved for who we are, not in spite of our imperfections but often because of them.

The sun now casts long shadows across the grass, a visual metaphor for the day's end—and yet I feel an inner sunrise, a burgeoning warmth that speaks of new beginnings and possibilities. I rise from the bench, my heart full with an introspective peace and a hopeful outlook. The trials I've faced, the luck that has graced my path, they haven't just fortified me; they've compelled me to extend a hand to those still struggling.

"Time to go," I murmur to myself, stepping off the well-worn path and into the embrace of the evening. The world is vast, filled with untold stories, pain, and beauty, and as I move forward, I carry with me the unwavering belief in resilience and redemption. For after every storm, there is calm. After every night, a dawn. And for every person who feels lost, there is a way back home—to hope, to life, to love.

As I sit on the edge of my bed, staring into the twilight that filters through the blinds, my mind churns with memories. There's a quietness inside me, a reflective pool collecting the rain of past experiences. I've had to confront many storms, some of my own making. Regrets? Yes, I have a few. Yet in acknowledging my missteps, I find a path to forgive myself, understanding that each one has been a stone upon which I've built the man I am today.

The echoes of a challenging childhood still linger in the corners of my being. Poverty wasn't just a word; it was the walls that confined me, the empty plates, the threadbare clothes. But it was more than material lack—it was the absence of security. The sting of harsh words and harder hands left marks deeper than bruises. A fever once claimed me, its scarlet fingers pulling me away from life's embrace, if only for a moment. On that living room couch, I brushed against eternity, yet somehow I was pulled back—a second chance granted by fate or fortune, carrying with me a message from an unknown figure in the light. "You have much to do yet, Bobby. Your father awaits you. It's time to return."

I've tumbled headlong into danger more times than I care to count. Once, gravity beckoned as I plunged over a hundred feet into a ravine, a jumble of logs and rocks awaiting below. The adrenaline surged, a wild rush of terror and exhilaration. But when the dust settled and silence returned, I stood, remarkably unscathed. It was as if the universe itself blinked in surprise, refusing to let me go that easily. Was it an angel that guided me safely to the floor of that ravine as my mother believes? Or was it the pure luck of the kid called Mr. Magoo that caused me to land safely on the shores of that stream?

With a boyish fearlessness—or maybe ignorance—I once pedaled hard toward the sky, launching my bike and myself off the roof of my house. Gravity won that round, but only the bike bore the scars. And there were those electric towers, tall silhouettes against the sky, their danger as clear as the warning signs that surrounded them. But climb them I did, heart pounding, every rung a dare to the fates that watched.

Mr. Magoo, they called me, after the cartoon character who walked blindly through chaos, untouched by the mayhem around him. There was laughter in the nickname, but beneath it, an acknowledgment of the incredible luck that seemed to follow me. Runaway trains, too, joined the list of harrowing adventures, each escape adding another layer to the legend I never sought to write.

These moments, these brushes with fate, are threads in the tapestry of my existence. Each close call, each miraculous survival, has become a testament to an unseen strength, a resilience that I can't claim as solely my own. Looking back, I can see the invisible hands—

perhaps destiny, divine intervention, or sheer dumb luck—that have guided me through.

Now, as the day gives way to night, I realize that the darkness isn't a void but a canvas. It waits for the dawn to paint new beginnings, fresh opportunities to rise again, to face the challenges that await. My journey is far from over; it's a road marked with the signs of trials and triumphs alike.

The hope that springs eternal within me is not born of naiveté. It's forged in the fires of adversity, quenched in the waters of reflection. I am a living testament to the power of hope, to the possibility of redemption, to the indomitable human spirit that refuses to be extinguished.

I rise from the bed, my thoughts shifting from the past to the present, to the future. In the mirror, I catch a glimpse of the boy who survived his upbringing, the young man who defied gravity, and the older, wiser soul who sees life's value in every breath. With each step forward, I carry the lessons of yesterday, the gratitude for today, and the hope for tomorrow.

"Let's see what you have in store for me," I whisper to the world, ready to embrace whatever comes next, knowing that no matter how fiercely the wind may blow, I will bend but never break. After all, I am Bobby Quayle—survivor, dreamer, believer in second chances—and this is my story.

The morning sun was barely rising, its first rays touching the edge of my bedroom curtains as I slipped out of bed. My feet found the familiar coldness of the floorboards beneath them, a stark contrast to the warmth of the covers I'd just abandoned. It was in these quiet moments, before the rest of the world stirred, that my mind would wander down the rugged path of my past.

I walked over to the window, fingers tracing the fabric of the curtain before pulling it back gently. The light spilled into the room, casting long shadows that seemed to carry the weight of the memories I held. Divorce had struck me twice; the pain and disarray felt like wild brushfires that consumed everything in their paths. The first time, it swept through my life with a ferocity that left nothing but scorched earth. Mary's departure came like a thief in the night, taking not just the love we shared but leaving a trail of betrayal in its wake.

Later, bankruptcy followed—once with Ricky-Bobby's deceitful business practices, then again when market forces beyond my control tore through our finances like a tornado. Each time, I watched helplessly as the life I had built crumbled, brick by brick, until I was knee-deep in the rubble of broken dreams and promises.

But the scars were not only financial or emotional. A sharp twinge in my upper back serves as a physical reminder of the cost of service to my country—a sacrifice encapsulated by a moment when the ground met my body in an unforgiving embrace. My fellow soldiers became ghosts in my life, whispers that turned away from my injury-induced vulnerability.

In the silence of those days, I mourned a father I never knew, his absence a hollow echo that resonated through the years. And Mandy, my loyal companion, whose trusting eyes looked up at me one last time before I made the heartbreaking decision to ease her suffering. These losses clustered together in a short span, relentless waves crashing over me.

Yet here I stood, gazing out at the dawn of a new day. The resilience that had carried me through every hardship didn't come from blind luck or some inexhaustible well of strength. It was born from each fall, each failure—lessons learned and wisdom earned.

My mother, Elaine, with her quiet fortitude, has instilled in me the understanding that adversity is not a roadblock but a stepping stone. Cheryl, ever my anchor, offered a love that weathered every storm. Bernd's laughter echoed in my head, a reminder that joy could be found even amid chaos. And Sergeant Martinez's unwavering support proved comradeship transcended the uniform.

As I stood there, I realized how every piece fit together, forging the person I had become. The victories and the defeats, the joys and the sorrows, they had molded me, shaped me into someone who could withstand the gusts of fate and still stand tall.

My reflection in the glass showed the lines of time etched upon my face, but within my eyes burned a fire undiminished by the years.

I couldn't change the past nor did I wish to. Each moment was a brushstroke in the vivid painting of my life.

"Today is another chance," I murmured to myself, a mantra of hope for what lay ahead. With a deep breath, I let the curtain fall back into place and turned away from the window, ready to step into the uncertainty of the future, carrying the certainty of my past triumphs and tribulations like armor.

For in this journey, I am both the traveler and the mapmaker, and while the destination may be unknown, the path is rich with possibility. So with a heart full of hope and a spirit attuned to the rhythm of perseverance, I embrace the day, steadfast in the belief that no matter how fierce the storm, the sun always rises again.

My fingers grazed the chipped paint of the park bench, the cool morning air cloaking the city in a soft mist. Here I was, sitting alone amid the whispers of dawn, surrounded by silent witnesses to my solitude—the rustling trees, the empty swings swaying gently as if moved by unseen children from days gone by. The sun hadn't yet broken the horizon, but its promise lingered in the periphery of a purpling sky.

I came here often to reflect, to breathe, to gather the scattered pieces of myself and fit them back together before the world awakened. Each day was a testament to survival, a new page in my unwritten autobiography that chronicled not just my existence, but my persistence.

"Life's punches come hard and fast," I thought, remembering Rocky's words. They had resonated with me since childhood, embedding themselves deep within my psyche, a mantra for the battles I'd face. "The world ain't all sunshine and rainbows." That line had been a shadow accompanying each step I took through the valleys of my life.

I recalled the sting of betrayal, the cacophony of heartbreak, the cold isolation in the barracks after my injury. It would have been easy to lie there on the ground of despair, to let the weight of the world pin me down indefinitely. But each time, somehow, I found the strength to rise—a little more bruised, perhaps, but unbroken.

The bench felt hard against my back, a reminder of reality's unyielding nature. But like this bench, I was steadfast. I'd gotten hit, harder than I ever imagined. Yet here I was, still moving forward, still taking it.

"Everything happens for a reason," I whispered to the morning, to the city of Berea, to myself. It wasn't an excuse or a dismissal. It was an acknowledgment of the intricate tapestry woven by each joy and each adversity I had faced.

Cheryl believed that too, her faith never wavering. She saw the design when I could only see tangled threads. Elaine, with her quiet strength born from years of solo battles, knew the resilience that was demanded of us. And Bernd…he'd always joked about my nine lives, but I knew he understood the earnestness of the struggle.

As light began to seep into the day, washing over buildings and streets with gentle hues, a sense of purpose swelled within me. Today would be filled with decisions, some small, others monumental. But regardless of their size, they would be mine to make, mine to own.

"Life will beat you to your knees if you let it." I stood up from the bench, feeling the truth of these words in every fiber of my being. It wasn't about avoiding the hits—that was impossible. It was about enduring them, absorbing them, allowing them to propel me forward instead of knocking me back.

I walked away from the bench, my footsteps resolute on the path ahead. There were moments I wished I could erase, choices I regretted. But those regrets had shaped me too, sharpened my edges, honed my resolve.

"Today is another chance," I affirmed, stepping into the burgeoning daylight. With every sunrise, there was hope, an opportunity to write another line in my story—a story marked by scars, yes, but also by endless possibilities.

And so I kept moving forward because that's how winning is done.

CHAPTER 21

HAVE FAITH AND
NEVER GIVE UP!

I lace up my walking shoes in the hush of early morning, the darkness still clinging to the edges of the sky. The road ahead is quiet, a blank canvas awaiting the brushstrokes of dawn. As I start my walk, the rhythmic thud of my footsteps becomes a meditation, each step a testament to my journey.

Far better is it to dare mighty things, Roosevelt's words echo in my thoughts. They've been a beacon for me, illuminating the path through the fog of uncertainty. It's not just about the victories; it's about the audacity to reach for them despite the fear of failure.

My breaths come in steady puffs, visible in the cool air, as I push myself up the incline that I once avoided, back when fear held more sway over my choices. But now I chase the hill with a fervor, hungry for its challenge. "To win glorious triumphs," I remind myself, even if those triumphs are as simple as conquering this daily climb.

The first light of day begins to spill over the horizon, painting the sky with strokes of pink and orange. It's a masterpiece of possibility, a reminder that each new day brings its own set of chances to dream big. And with each dream, there's a leap of faith—an act of trust in something greater than myself and in the strength I've found within.

"Have faith" becomes a mantra that propels me forward, synchronizing with my heartbeat. I think of Cheryl, her steadfast belief in us, and how her love has been a compass through every storm; my mother's resilience, woven into my DNA, a tapestry of survival and grit; Bernd's laughter, a reminder that joy can be found even in the midst of trials.

As the top of the hill comes into view, my legs burn with the effort, but so does something deeper inside me—the fire of determination, kindled by years of getting back up, dusting off, and moving forward. I crest the hill and pause to catch my breath, looking out at the world awakening below.

"Even though checkered by failure." I let out a breath, watching it mingle with the crisp morning air. Failure is a part of the landscape, a necessary contrast that makes success all the brighter. I've known its bitter taste, but it has only made the sweetness of achievement more profound.

The descent is easier, a time to gather thoughts and strength for whatever lies ahead. "Because they live in a gray twilight that knows not victory nor defeat." I refuse to dwell in the shadows of what could have been. My life has been painted with bold colors—some dark, some brilliant, but all part of a larger work that is uniquely mine.

With the sun fully risen, casting long shadows behind me, I make my way home. There's a promise in that golden light—a pact between the universe and those daring enough to heed its call. Today, like every day, I'll choose to be one of the daring, to keep trying, no matter the odds.

"Keep trying," I whisper as I open the door to the warmth of my home, the smell of fresh coffee greeting me. A new day awaits, full of might-have-beens, and I am ready to meet it head-on. Because that's how winning is done.

To anyone who may be reading this, if my personal recollections have in any way touched your heart or helped you reevaluate a permanent decision, please know that you have given my words a purpose beyond measure. I am grateful beyond words for the chance to share my story with you, and I hope you continue to read on as I reveal how my life has been transformed from that dark day when I nearly gave up everything.

This book's value cannot be measured in currency; its true worth lies in the possibility that it may ignite a spark of hope within someone who is lost and struggling. I would be honored to meet you, to hear your own story of courage and resilience in the face of adversity. Please reach out to me at Quaymar@gmail.com. Your experience is just as valuable as mine, and together, our stories can shine a light for those still wandering in darkness, searching for their own ray of hope. Let us join hands and lift each other up toward the bright future that awaits us all.

CHAPTER 22

BONUS
A DREAM ACHIEVED

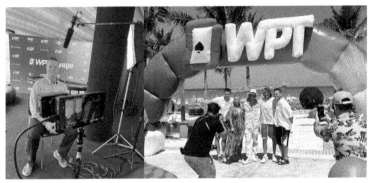

Me being interviewed on camera about the book and experience on
the Voyage. On the right, the stars of the WPT at Bimini Beach.

As I mentioned earlier in this book, one of my bucket list items was
to win my way into a major televised poker tournament. As fate
would have it, I have done just that as this book was being edited
by the professionals at Covenant Books. I also mentioned that my
happy ending is yet unwritten, and because the timing allows me
to add this bonus chapter, I feel compelled to share it in this book
because, yes…Mr. Magoo strikes again! Please read on to learn how
this happy ending just keeps getting better and how, perhaps, I am
being guided by fate once again.

*****

I'm sitting here in the dim glow of the airport terminal, the hum of distant conversations and the occasional rumble of a taking-off plane providing a familiar yet surreal backdrop to the moment. My flight to Miami is just an hour away from boarding, but my mind is not on the journey ahead; it's still reeling with the reality that I've achieved something I never thought possible.

A crumpled boarding pass rests in my hands, and every so often, I smooth out its edges, as if to convince myself it's real. This piece of paper is more than just a ticket; it's proof of a dream turning into tangible success. A major poker event awaits me at the end of this flight, one that I've won my way into against all odds.

Looking back, I can't help but think about the turns my life has taken. The road has been anything but straight, riddled with potholes and detours that tested my spirit and resolve. But as I sit here, it strikes me how each of those trials was a step leading to this very seat in this bustling terminal.

"Everything happens for a reason," I whisper to myself, a mantra that has become my lifeline through the darkest hours. There's light at the end of the tunnel—I'm proof of that. And it's a bright, blinding, beautiful light that promises blessings beyond imagination for those who dare to keep faith, to persevere no matter how unforgiving the path might seem.

Rocky Balboa's words echo in my mind, a motivational speech that feels like it was tailor-made for me: "It's not about how hard you can hit. It's about how hard you can *get* hit and keep moving forward. That's how winning is done!" How many times have I replayed that line in my head? How many times have those words picked me up off the canvas of life?

I've taken hits, more than I care to count; but here I am, still standing, still moving forward. I've learned that resilience isn't about not feeling the pain or the doubt; it's about acknowledging them and deciding to take another step anyway. It's about being hopeful, about finding that sliver of chance and grasping it with both hands.

In the reflection of the large windows overlooking the runway, I catch a glimpse of myself. Short-cropped brown hair, more salt than pepper now, frames a face that's seen its share of struggles. But it's the eyes that hold the story—they're the eyes of a man who knows what it's like to be down but not out, a man who's slow to trust the hand he's dealt but plays it with all he's got.

An announcement breaks through my thoughts, a gentle reminder that my flight will soon begin boarding. I stand up, stretching limbs that feel suddenly energized by the prospect of what lies ahead. After tucking the boarding pass safely in my pocket, I shoulder my bag and take a deep breath.

"Here we go," I say to myself, a smile creeping across my face. You see, I've come to understand that the game of life, much like poker, is about playing the hand you're dealt to the best of your ability. And sometimes, just sometimes, that's enough to win your way into paradise.

The cards fan out before my eyes, an intricate dance of red and black, a language I've come to speak fluently in the quiet hours of my newfound freedom. *Retirement*, a word that once echoed with the hollowness of uncertainty, now thrums with the vitality of opportunity. My fingers, steady from years of navigating life's unpredictable currents, riffle through pages of strategy and probability—poker books stacked like sentinels of knowledge on my desk at home.

"Passengers for flight 237 to Miami, please begin boarding at gate 12."

The announcement nudges me back to the present, the airport bustling around me—a hive of comings and goings, each person a story, a journey, a dream waiting to unfold. I rise, the weight of anticipation a pleasant burden on my shoulders. A hobby once cradled in the margins of my life has unfurled into a pursuit that fuels me, igniting a spark I thought had long dimmed.

I remember the first time I watched Chris Moneymaker's triumph, his name predestined for greatness, etching itself into history. It was a revelation—the everyman conquering the titans of the felt. And there I was, rooted to my couch, heart thundering as if those hands were my own.

"Sir, are you traveling to Miami?" The voice is polite, tinged with the robotic cadence of someone who has asked this question too many times today.

I nod, a smile tugging at my lips. "Yes, yes, I am."

"Please have your boarding pass ready," she replies, her gaze already moving past me to the next in line.

I obediently hold the crisp paper in my hand, a symbol of what's to come. In my peaceful retirement, I have found both comfort and excitement on the virtual battlefield, where kings and queens reign supreme, and aces can be either victory or defeat. Through online courses and advice from experienced players through headphones, my instincts have been honed and my determination sharpened. And then there's ClubWPT—my digital arena—where I've fought against opponents without ever seeing their faces, as their strategies remain hidden behind screen names and avatars, all in pursuit of cash prizes and entry into prestigious championship tournaments around the world.

A single card can change everything. Isn't that the truth of life as well? One decision, one chance encounter, one bold move—that's all it takes to alter the course of our narrative. As I step forward, my footfalls resonate with the quiet confidence of countless hands played, lessons learned, and risks taken.

Luck, they say, is the residue of design, and perhaps they're right. But I like to think there's more to it than that. It's about seeing the odds and daring to dream beyond them. It's about resilience, about acknowledging them and deciding to take another step anyway. It's about being hopeful, about finding that sliver of chance and grasping it with both hands.

The humid air embraces me the moment I step out of the Uber, a stark contrast to the sterile chill of the airport terminal I have left behind. The Miami sun is a golden orb suspended in a cloudless sky as I make my way toward the port. My heart thrums with anticipation; today is not just another day; it's the beginning of an adventure I never saw coming.

I join the throng of passengers at the port, each one a character in their own story but all converging for this unique chapter at sea. The wait is long, teeming with unforeseen delays that test one's patience, but it gives me time to reflect on how far I've come. From evenings spent poring over poker books to countless online tournaments, every fold, every bet, and every bluff has led me here.

"Boarding is now open," comes the announcement, and like a floodgate released, we surge forward. The ship looms before us, grand and imposing—a floating calusari of dreams and possibilities. I step onto the vessel, my senses alight with the scent of the ocean mingled with fresh paint and anticipation.

Before I can even acquaint myself with the polished decks and lavish surroundings, my phone vibrates with unexpected urgency. An alert flashes across the screen—an invitation to a private party on the sixteenth deck. My breath catches in my throat. This is no ordinary welcome aboard; it's an exclusive gathering of the World Poker Tour's luminaries.

As the elevator ascends, each ding marking our progress skyward, a smile plays upon my lips. It isn't just about being amid the stars of the WPT—Lynn Gilmartin's grace, Matt Savage—The Crooner, Tony Dunst's sharp wit, Vince Van Patten's amiable presence; it's about being recognized as part of something greater than myself.

The doors slide open, revealing the vibrant thrum of conversation and laughter. I step out, feeling like a small-town hero stepping onto the big stage for the first time. There they are: the faces I know so well from TV screens, now animated and real, only an arm's length away.

"Welcome, Bobby!" Lynn greets me with a warmth that feels like a sunrise, dispelling any shadows of doubt. "We're thrilled to have you join us."

"Thank you," I manage, my voice steady even though my heart is racing. This is more than just a game; it's a symbol of life's unexpected turns—the hands we're dealt and how we choose to play them.

I find myself gazing out over the railings, the ocean stretching in infinite directions. This vast blue expanse is like the future— unpredictable and mysterious but also inviting. And at this moment, buoyed by an ocean of hope and surrounded by fellow Streamers, I can't help but feel lucky. I finally have the privilege of meeting some fellow Stream Team members in person, such as Fundamit and her awesome and kind husband, RichAl63, both formidable opponents at the tables. Then there's Metajohnm and INFIN8, both outstanding players and all-around nice guys, to name but a few. I also had the distinct privilege of meeting Jeremy Clemons, the man responsible for our amazing experiences online on ClubWPT.

"Here's to new beginnings," I whisper to the wind, letting the words carry off into the horizon. This cruise isn't just a path to potential glory at the poker table; it's a reminder that life itself is the grandest gamble, and I'm all in.

As I mingle through the private party, the clinking of glasses and laughter creating a symphony of what I'd call pure joy, I feel a tug on my arm. Turning around, I notice Michael, one of the World Poker Tour representatives. He was tuned into our WPT Stream Team chat some time ago where I had casually mentioned my book—a labor of love born from countless trials and a testament to resilience.

"Your story sounds intriguing, Bobby," Michael says. "Melissa, our producer, would like to know more about your journey. Could be inspiring for many."

My heart skips a beat. The mere fact that someone from the WPT is taking an interest in my story feels surreal. I gaze around the room, trying to locate Melissa in the crowd. I turn to Michael. There he is, his friendly eyes meeting mine over the rim of his drink, a kind smile on his bearded face, which makes me feel instantly at ease. His approachable demeanor stands in stark contrast to the opulence surrounding us, a reminder that real wealth lies in human connection.

"Hey, Bobby!" Michael calls out as he navigates his way toward me, his hand extended in a gesture of friendship. "Melissa can't wait to hear about your book."

"Thank you, Michael," I reply, shaking his hand. His grip is firm, reassuring. "I'm just...overwhelmed by all this."

"Good things happen when you least expect them," he says with a chuckle, his voice carrying the wisdom of someone who has seen the world but never lost touch with the simple joys of life.

"Seems like it," I agree, my eyes briefly scanning the deck—stars of the poker universe laughing and talking, the night sky above us, an ocean of possibilities. This is more than a gathering; it's a celebration of chance and skill, of fortunes won and lost, each person here bonded by their love of the game.

"Let's make sure we catch up later," Michael adds before returning to the festivities, leaving me to ponder his words and share my story with Melissa.

The evening wears on, a tapestry of shared stories and laughter, the camaraderie among the Stream Team family palpable. Michael has unwittingly set in motion a series of events that exceeded all my expectations. It seems that every conversation and handshake is a step toward something bigger, a new chapter waiting to be written. And throughout it all, there is Melissa—professional amid the revelry, her genuine interest in my tale a beacon of hope.

I lean against the rail, looking out at the sea. Each wave that breaks against the ship's hull whispers of destiny, of paths converging and diverging in the grand design of life. At this moment, surrounded by the kindness of strangers who are quickly becoming friends, I feel humbled—like a lone sailor navigating by the stars, finding his way home.

"Life," I muse silently, "is the ultimate poker game. And maybe, just maybe, I'm holding a winning hand."

The rhythmic hum of the ship's engine resonates with my own heartbeat as I stand near the poker tables, the felt surface an arena for the mind. The chips clink like a chorus of decision and consequence, a symphony I'm about to join. Melissa's words from earlier echo in my thoughts: an interview about my life, my struggles, my book— on camera. The gravity of her offer anchors me to a reality I have never dared to envision.

I clasp my hands together, feeling the warmth of anticipation mingled with the cool resolve that has seen me through life's tempests. This opportunity is more than a spotlight; it's a lighthouse guiding the lost ships of souls who may find solace in my story. With each passing second, the once-distant hope of sharing my journey grows tangible, the texture of possibility against my skin.

"Mr. Quayle, your table is ready," a staff member announces, pulling me back into the present.

"Thank you," I mutter, my voice steady despite the whirlwind of thoughts.

As I take my seat among the competitors, the familiar rush of adrenaline courses through me, a silent ally whispering strategies and patience. Around me, faces etched with focus and determination reflect my own inner fire, each player seeking their moment of triumph.

The cards are dealt, one hand after another, a dance of chance and skill. The tournament progresses, and with each fallen adversary, the vision of the final table becomes clearer, closer. It's not just about the game anymore; it's about proving to myself that the resilience woven through my past has merit, that it can propel me toward new heights.

And then there it is—the final table. My hands don't tremble as I stack my chips, nor does my heart falter. Instead, a quiet pride settles over me. To have come this far, from the depths of despair to sitting among the top contenders, is a testament to something greater than luck. It's a testament to the enduring spirit that has carried me through life's darkest corridors.

Perhaps this is the moment that will redefine what's possible. As I look around at the remaining players, a sense of camaraderie envelopes us. We are all warriors of fate in our own right, each with a story, each with a dream.

"Nice hand," I compliment an opponent after a particularly tense showdown. The mutual respect is palpable, an unspoken language of the tables.

I allow myself to imagine, just for an instant, what it would be like to embrace the title of semipro. Another dream, another mountain to climb. But isn't that what life's about? To keep moving forward, reaching for those peaks that seem insurmountable?

"Play your best, Bobby," I silently encourage myself. "Let this be the hand that writes a new chapter."

And whether or not I hold the winning cards, I know one thing for certain: I have already won. For in finding the courage to share my story, to inspire even one person to persevere, I have achieved the greatest victory of all.

The sun casts a golden glow over the azure waters as I sit at the poker table, cards in hand, my mind racing with strategies and possibilities. The clinking of chips blends harmoniously with the distant laughter and splashing from the pool deck above. Each day has been a whirlwind of activity, a cascade of moments that blur together into an exhilarating dream.

I have found myself, a man who has seen the darker side of life, basking in the unexpected warmth of success. The cash games treat me kindly, swelling my wallet and feeding the flames of a newfound confidence within me. Tournament after tournament, I hold my own, watch pots slide my way, and feel the curious eyes of strangers appraising my play. My heart swells with every victory, and even in defeat, I find lessons to be learned.

It is on one such afternoon, under the benevolent gaze of the tropical sun, that I reflect on the journey that has brought me here. I remember the times when hope seemed like a distant star, shimmering but forever out of reach. Yet now here I am, holding on to that star, its light infusing my life with a radiance I never thought possible. Gratitude washes over me, a silent prayer of thanks escaping my lips for the decision I made years ago to keep fighting when surrender seemed the only option.

Then comes the day of the interview—the culmination of so many serendipitous events. Nerves flutter in my stomach like a flock of restless birds as I approach the designated area. The crew bustles around, adjusting lighting and testing equipment, their professionalism a stark contrast to the leisurely pace of the cruise.

"Mr. Quayle, we're ready for you," calls a voice, snapping me back to reality.

I nod, steeling myself, and take a seat as directed. The cold touch of the microphone clip against my skin reminds me this is all very real. Bright lights focus on me, creating an island of visibility amid the shadowy expanse of the room.

"Remember, just be yourself," I murmur, taking a deep breath. The camera lens stares at me, an unblinking eye waiting to capture my story.

As the questions begin, I speak from the heart. My words are not just sounds in the air; they are fragments of my soul, my experiences—my truth. I talk about the highs and lows, the resilience it takes to weather the storms, and the incredible fortune I've found in a game of chance. My voice may have wavered, but my spirit stand firm.

"Cut! That was excellent, Bobby," the interviewer says, offering a smile that holds both encouragement and respect.

With the interview concluded and the lights dimming, I feel a peculiar sensation—an odd mix of relief and exhilaration. I have shared parts of my life that once I would've locked away, and now they are free, floating into the world to perhaps land in the hearts of those who need them most.

I linger there for a moment, alone with my thoughts, feeling like someone who has stepped out of obscurity and into a spotlight I never sought but somehow earned. I allow myself to bask in the surreal sense that I, Bobby Quayle, am momentarily a celebrity not for fame or glory but for simply being a man who refused to give up.

"Thank you," I whisper quietly not to anyone in particular but to the universe, to fate, to whatever divine force guided me to this point. "Thank you for this chance to shine, even if just for a while."

And as I walk away from the set, the weight of the microphone pack lifted from my shoulders, I know that no matter what the future holds, this moment—this incredible, unexpected journey—is a beacon of hope, proof that sometimes life deals you the winning hand when you least expect it.

The cards fan out before me, their faces a blur of numbers and suits. The turn has been kind, and the river even more so. But as I place my hand on the felt, eights full of nines, I see it—the flicker of triumph in my opponent's eyes. Then he lays down his hand, nines full of eights, an implausible coup that sends my chips sliding across the table.

"Cut!" the director calls out. "That's perfect, Bobby!"

I sit there, stunned for a moment, the sting of the bad beat still fresh. Yet it's all part of the show. The film crew buzzes around me, capturing every angle, every emotion. This isn't just poker; this is life encapsulated in a game—an allegory of the rises and falls that mark my journey.

With only two 1,000 chips left, I feel a familiar resilience stir within me. Pushing back against despair with practiced ease, I steady my gaze, ready to rebuild. And rebuild I do. Through calculated risks and steadfast composure, I claw my way back into the game, chip by chip, until my stack towers over 30,000 once again. It's a testament to the philosophy that has carried me through darker times: when you're at your lowest, the only way is up.

The crew has since moved on to other assignments. But it isn't just about the tables anymore. They film me elsewhere too, like on the sunlit deck, watching people play pickleball with an intensity that matches any high-stakes game. They capture me strolling along the beach, the sun setting behind me, casting long shadows on the sand, my thoughts turning like the tide to the blessings and trials that have shaped me.

"Action, Bobby," Melissa, the producer, prompts.

"Thanks to ClubWPT, I have won my way into paradise, and so can *you!*" I declare, pointing directly at the camera with a new-found sense of purpose.

"That's money!" Melissa exclaims, her affirmation sending a ripple of pride through me.

As the crew packs away their equipment, the last light of day fading from the sky, I can't help but reflect on the surreal nature of it all. Here I am, a man who once felt invisible to the world, now standing in front of bright lights, sharing my tale of persistence and luck. It's a stark reminder that sometimes the most extraordinary opportunities arise from the simplest acts of courage—like entering a poker tournament or opening up about one's struggles.

"Trust me, if I can do it, anyone can," I murmur to myself, the words resonating deep within. That phrase isn't just for the commercial; it's a mantra for life, a call to action for anyone teetering on the brink of giving up.

As I walk away from the spotlight, the ocean breeze brushes against my skin, whispering secrets of hope and chance. I'm no longer just Bobby Quayle; I'm a beacon of what can be achieved with a little faith and a lot of heart. And maybe, just maybe, my story can light the way for others searching for their own path to paradise.

As the final echoes of laughter and applause from the film crew fade into the background, I find myself standing alone, enveloped in the afterglow of a day that will forever be etched in my memory. The sun has dipped below the horizon, painting the sky with streaks of pink and orange, a backdrop so vivid it almost seems as if the heavens themselves are celebrating my fortune.

I gather my thoughts, ready to retreat to solitude, when Dave, the sound guy whose steady hands mic'd me up for the commercial, approaches with a companion by his side. Her name is Nadine, and she's wearing the kind of genuine smile that instantly puts you at ease. He introduces us, and her eyes sparkle with a writer's curiosity—the same curiosity that drove me to pen down my own life's trials and triumphs.

"Your story, Bobby... It moved me," Nadine confesses, her voice carrying the warm timbre of someone who has spent a lifetime listening to others. "It's not just about poker. It's about survival, about hope."

Those words, so simple yet profound, wrap around me like a comforting shawl. We speak briefly, sharing the kinship that only fellow writers can understand—the need to translate life into words that heal, inspire, and connect.

Then, as naturally as the tide meets the shore, Nadine shares her connection to an organization close to her heart—an organization striving to prevent suicide among our military heroes. And as fate would have it, her son (a two-star general no less) stands at the helm of this noble cause. My pulse quickens at the serendipity of it all, at the thought of my book finding its way to those who may see their reflection in my struggles and find the strength to persevere.

"Would you reach out to him?" she suggests, hope underlining every syllable. "He could really use your insight."

The promise of making even the smallest difference in the lives of our service members, those brave souls who often bear invisible scars, ignites something within me. This is more than a fortuitous encounter—it's a calling.

"Absolutely, Nadine. It would be my honor," I reply, the gravity of the opportunity settling deep in my bones.

We exchange contact information, and as we part ways, the cool night air whispers of new beginnings. I stroll along the now-quiet deck, the gentle sway of the ship a soothing rhythm beneath my feet. The stars above wink at me, cosmic spectators to the unfolding chapter of my life.

Fortune smiles upon me when I find myself in the right place at the right time, granting me the esteemed privilege of speaking with Nadine's son, Air Force Major General Ed "Hertz" Vaughan. He has a keen interest in my story, and he graciously introduces me to his dear friend General Doug "Odie" Slocum. As a published author himself, his book *Violent Positivity* comes highly recommended by yours truly—not only a riveting tale of an American hero but also a treasure trove of wise advice that showcases the power of positive thinking.

But wait, there's more!

My heart races as I stare in disbelief at the computer screen. Against all odds, as I work on the final edit of this book, I have secured not one but two coveted seats, valued at $1,100 each, in a major World Poker Tour Tournament thanks to ClubWPT! And not just any tournament but one that will be held in the dazzling lights and high-stakes environment of Las Vegas this December. The rush of adrenaline surges through my veins as I imagine facing off against some of the best poker players in the world, with millions of dollars on the line. This, like the WPT Poker Championship Voyage, is another moment I've been waiting for my entire life! Thank you, Jesus!

As I put the finishing touches on my edits, a feeling of fulfillment washes over me. My fellow poker player and stream team member, Onerenegade, has reached out to share his thoughts on my book and its subject matter. His words bring tears to my eyes as he reveals how it has given him strength to keep fighting his battle against cancer. He is a warrior, and I pray for him every day, hoping that my book can continue to be a source of inspiration and support for him in his time of need.

And so, dear readers, I humbly share these words with you not to boast but as a testament to the indomitable spirit that resides within us all. The journey ahead may still be unwritten, but as I stand here today, I am living proof of the incredible potential that lies within each one of us—hope, resilience, and perhaps just a sprinkling of good fortune.

If my story has reached you, touched a chord within your soul, know that it's a melody we can all sing. Reach out to Quaymar@gmail.com, share your tale, and let us walk this path together. For in the end, it's the shared stories of our hardships and victories that bind us, that remind us to choose life, to keep fighting, to never surrender to despair.

Best wishes, and God bless you on your journey. May you always find the light amid the shadows, and may you too discover the paradise that awaits beyond the trials.

EPILOGUE

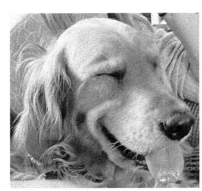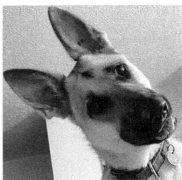

As I sat by the pond in our backyard, the sound of the waterfall murmured in agreement with my every contemplative thought. The fire before me crackled and hissed as I stirred the hot coals, sending a shower of sparks into the twilight sky—a miniature galaxy born from the embers. With deliberate care, I placed another log onto the fire; it was a small act, yet it felt like fueling the very essence of our home's warmth.

A few yards away, Molly and Reagan tumbled through the grass in an enthusiastic display of canine joy. They were golden and black streaks against the green, their playful barks punctuating the serene evening air. Watching them, a gentle smile crept across my face. They didn't need much to be happy—just an open field and each other's company.

Cheryl, the embodiment of patience and love, had claimed her usual spot on the wooden bench I'd fashioned with my own hands years ago. She watched the flames dance, their light casting a soft glow on her features. A cigarette rested between her fingers, the smoke curling upwards before dissipating into nothingness—a stark contrast to the permanence of the bond we shared.

I glanced over at her, the woman who had become my lighthouse in storms I never thought I'd survive. "Honey," I began, my voice steady but imbued with the weight of a thousand unspoken words, "I want you to know that you and your amazing daughters, and grandson are part of my happy ending, most of which hasn't even been written yet."

Beneath the veil of night, the world around us seemed to hold its breath. There was a sacred feeling in the air, as if the universe itself recognized the gravity of a soul laid bare.

"Everything I see here—the dogs, our house, the cars, even the bank accounts and investments—it's all part of my reward for choosing to live on that day when I nearly gave in to despair." The declaration hung between us, not a plea for validation but a testament to a life once fractured now made whole.

The truth was Cheryl and her daughters had given me more than just a second chance; they had given me a reason to redefine what it meant to be alive. Every challenge faced, every obstacle overcome, had led me to this tranquil moment by the fire, where the simple act of living was no longer a burden but a gift.

In the end, it wasn't the material possessions that held value—it was the laughter, the shared silences, the collective strength when one of us faltered. It was the understanding that while pain might be a chapter, it would never be the entire story.

As the night deepened and the stars found their places above, I realized that hope wasn't just a fleeting sentiment; it was as resilient as the earth beneath our feet, as boundless as the skies stretching overhead. And with Cheryl by my side, the unwritten pages of our lives hold endless possibilities.

The cool evening breeze stirred the leaves around me, a subtle reminder of nature's persistent rhythm. I leaned back in my chair, my gaze drawn to the embers that glowed brighter with each gentle puff of wind. Watching the fire crackle and pop, I felt the warmth seep into my bones, chasing away the lingering chill of the past.

"Look at them," Cheryl murmured, her voice soft with affection as our dogs romped near the water's edge, their carefree energy a stark contrast to the stillness that enveloped us. Molly leaped after a fluttering leaf while Reagan bounded beside her, both reveling in the simple joy of play.

A smile tugged at my lips. Over a decade ago, my world had been painted in shades of gray, a life devoid of the vibrant colors that now splashed across my days. Back then, loneliness had been my constant companion, the silence of an empty house echoing the hollowness within my chest.

But here, now, the symphony of life played a different tune. The laughter of my stepdaughters often filled the rooms, their vibrancy and youth a balm to my weary soul. They'd welcomed me with open arms, allowing me to step into a role I'd never imagined for myself—a father figure, a guiding hand, a source of unwavering support.

And then there is our grandson, a tiny miracle who has reshaped our world yet again. His infectious giggles and wide-eyed wonder at the simplest things will undoubtedly remind me daily of how precious this second chance at life truly is.

"Can you believe it, Cheryl?" I said, the awe clear in my voice as I turned to face her. Her eyes met mine, a knowing smile playing on her lips as she took another drag from her cigarette, the orange glow briefly illuminating her features.

"Believe what, Bobby?" Her voice was a gentle prompt, laced with the patience of one who has seen the depths from which I'd climbed.

"That we're here," I began, my voice thick with emotion. "That life... It's so much more than I ever thought it could be, after all the darkness."

Cheryl reached out, her hand finding mine, an anchor in the memories that threatened to pull me under. "I always knew you had it in you to rise above it all," she whispered, her words a lifeline.

The love I held for this woman—it was boundless, having only grown stronger with time. She has become my haven, her daughters my unexpected blessings, and the life we are building together far surpasses the broken dreams of yesteryear.

In the quiet of the evening, surrounded by the tender embrace of family and the soft hum of nature, I marveled at the journey that had brought me here. The resilience that coursed through my veins wasn't just my own; it was a tapestry woven from the strength of those who stood beside me, those who believed in me when I struggled to believe in myself.

As the fire before us danced and swayed, I found solace in its unpredictable beauty. It was a reflection of life—wild, untamed, and utterly breathtaking. With each flicker of flame, I was reminded that hope is not a mere whisper in the dark but a roar that echoes through the canyons of despair, lighting the way home.

"Every day is a gift," I murmured, the truth of the words settling deep within my soul. "A gift I'll never take for granted again."

Cheryl squeezed my hand, a silent affirmation that she shared my sentiment. Together, we watched the night unfold, the future an unwritten page that we would fill with stories of love, perseverance, and grace.

The home that encased this serene outdoor space was far removed from the modest abode of my past—a testament to the remarkable turn my life had taken. Now I resided in an upscale house nestled within a secluded development where the trees stood tall and the neighbors waved with genuine smiles. It was a stark contrast to the cramped quarters of my earlier years, where every creak of the floorboards told stories of struggle and uncertainty.

Mandy, my beloved dog who once shared my simpler life, had been a beacon of loyalty and love. Her intelligent eyes seemed to peer into my very soul, understanding the silent weight I carried. In her absence, Molly and Reagan had stepped into the role of faithful companions. They bore different names but carried the same spirit— intelligent and affectionate, they remind me daily of the bond that humans can forge with their four-legged friends.

Cheryl, her silhouette softened by the flickering flames, sat on the wooden bench I had crafted with my own hands long ago. She pulled gently on a cigarette, watching the embers soar skyward, her presence a quiet anchor in the fluidity of my reflections. The dogs' spirited play, the warmth of the fire, the contented sighs of cherished company—it all painted a picture so vividly different from the canvas of my life over a decade prior.

"Every crackle of this fire," I mused silently, "is like a note in the symphony of a life reborn." My gaze shifted to the dancing shadows cast upon Cheryl's face, the lines of time etched with grace and resilience. We didn't need words to communicate; our shared journey spoke volumes.

Resilience—that was the pulse of my story, the heartbeat that surged through the narrative of my existence. As I watched Molly chase Reagan around an ancient oak, their figures blending with the dusk, hope swelled within me. This was what it meant to overcome, to build anew from the ashes of despair.

In this tranquil moment, surrounded by the simple yet profound upgrades of my present reality, I felt a deep sense of gratitude. Life had been generous, not just in material blessings but in the opportunity to witness and savor such transformation. And as the night embraced us with its cool touch and the promise of dawn lingered just beyond the horizon, I knew that my story was far from over.

It was a tale still being written, each day a fresh page, and I was the author holding the pen. With introspection and hope as my guides, I would continue to craft a legacy not of what was lost but of what was found and cherished. And therein lay the true upgrade, the real luxury—living a life rich with purpose and love, no matter what the exterior might suggest.

The crackle of the fire was a soothing accompaniment to my thoughts as I added another log, watching sparks ascend like tiny beacons into the twilight sky. The scent of burning pine mingled with the earthy dampness rising from the pond's edge where I sat. Molly and Reagan bounded in the distance, their playful barks punctuating the evening's calm. Cheryl, my rock, exhaled a stream of smoke into the air, her gaze fixed on the hypnotic dance of the flames.

I leaned back, feeling the warmth of the fire against my skin, contrasting sharply with the cool breeze that swept over the yard. It was hard to believe there was a time when the cold grip of financial ruin had threatened to extinguish all hope. Back then, the economic collapse had ransacked my dreams, leaving me with nothing but the shell of a failed business and a bank account gasping for air. But here we were, years later, financially stable—a testament to resilience and the grace of second chances.

Cheryl has been instrumental in this turnaround, her tireless work blending seamlessly with the steady rhythm of my disability income and pension to create a safety net that now cradles our lives. Each paycheck she brings home is a stitch in the tapestry of her dedication to her daughters, woven with dedication and love. Her sacrifices have not gone unnoticed; they are the unsung verses of our shared song of perseverance.

And then there is the car—the sleek symbol of how far I have come. Where once an older model sedan sat, reluctant and weary in the driveway, now rests a luxury car that gleams under the garage lights like a trophy. Not one of vanity but of victory over life's unforeseen blows. It isn't just a mode of transport; it is a chariot that has risen from the ashes of despair, powered by faith and relentless will.

As the night deepened around us, I gazed at Cheryl, her features softened by the fire's glow. The material possessions were nice, sure, but they paled in comparison to the wealth of love and loyalty she represented. Together, we had weathered storms and emerged not just unscathed but stronger, our bond forged in adversity's relentless forge.

I felt the familiar twinge in my back, a reminder of the physical battles I'd endured, yet it did little to dampen my spirits. For I had learned that true wealth was not found in the balance of a bank account or the make of a car, but in the quiet moments of reflection by a pond, in the company of loyal dogs and a woman whose belief in me never wavered. It resided in the knowledge that no matter how battered we were by life's tempests, hope was our anchor and love our compass.

"Cheryl," I said softly, not wanting to disturb the peace, "I've come a long way, haven't I?"

She turned to me, a smile tugging at the corners of her mouth, her eyes reflecting the firelight and something deeper—perhaps the pride of shared triumphs. "Yes, Bobby, you certainly have."

With that affirmation, I looked up at the stars beginning to pepper the darkening canvas above, each one a distant beacon of possibility. Their steadfast light reminded me that even in the darkest times, there are pinpricks of hope waiting to be seen. And as long as we keep our gaze upward and our strides forward, the path ahead is bound to be illuminated by the unexpected joys of a life reclaimed.

The list of blessings—my life's stark transformation—is indeed endless. As I sit here, tending to the fire that has become a rite of reflection, I realize there is no need to enumerate further. The evidence of change surrounds me, palpable in every aspect of this very setting, from the tall trees that stand as silent witnesses to my resurgence, to the sturdy wooden bench, crafted by my own hands during a time when creating something tangible felt like a lifeline.

"Cheryl," I call softly, unable to keep the sense of wonder from my voice. She glances over from where she sits, her silhouette haloed by the flickering light. "We've built something incredible, haven't we?"

A quiet nod is all she offers, but it's enough—a testament to our incredible journeys that led us to each other late in life and found us here.

In those dark days, over a decade ago, I couldn't have envisioned this life. It was a time when the very act of breathing felt laborious, each day a mountain to climb with no summit in sight. But I persevered, I climbed, and somewhere along the way, the landscape changed.

Now I wake each morning not to dread but to possibility. Despite the chronic ache in my back—a constant reminder of past struggles—I find joy in the freedom that retirement affords me. Time, once an enemy that marched on with indifferent haste is now a friend, offering me the luxury to indulge in passions, to savor moments, to simply be.

I could go on for quite some time recounting the upgrades to my life since that fateful day when Jesus took the driver's seat, steering me away from despair. Carrie Underwood's lyrics, once a mere song on the radio, became a lifeline, echoing the sentiments of my soul until they were no longer just words but a catalyst.

My life today? It's better than I imagined it could ever be back then. Here I am, able to craft sentences and chapters, weaving my narrative into something tangible—that others might draw strength from my story. Writing this book, sharing these words, it's more than a task; it's my soul laid bare, a mosaic of pain and triumph.

Yes, I could list the material contrasts, the visible markers of a life improved. But what truly astounds me is the internal renovation—the peace that fills me, the gratitude that fuels me. These cannot be quantified or flaunted, yet they are my most precious acquisitions.

"Life is rich," I whisper to the night, to Cheryl, to myself. And as the stars emerge, dotting the sky with their resilient light, I know that each day is a canvas and hope the brush with which we paint our destinies.

The crackle of the fire was a symphony to my ears as the bright flames leapt into the twilight. I tossed another log onto the smoldering embers, watching them ignite with newfound vigor. It's mesmerizing how life can mirror such simple acts—how out of the remnants of what was, a spark can birth a blaze.

Molly and Reagan romped in the yard, their playful barks piercing the calm air. They chased each other, tails wagging, completely absorbed in their game—a reminder of the unconditional joy animals bring into our lives. I gave the pond a cursory glance, the water reflecting the last orange hues of the setting sun. The koi swam lazily, their scales glinting like liquid gold, and I felt a sense of accomplishment seeing the ecosystem I nurtured thrive.

My fingers itched for a pen, the urge to document this tranquility nearly overwhelming. There's a book laid open on my lap, half-filled with the ink of my reflections. I wonder if there are more books within me, more stories clamoring to be told. But for now, this narrative holds my focus—the story of redemption and hope that I'm determined to leave as my legacy.

Beyond the realm of words and pages, another passion calls to me—the strategic world of Texas Hold'em Poker. I've been honing my skills, calculating odds, and studying tells, preparing for a battle of wits on the green felt battlegrounds. The World Championship of Poker looms on my horizon, a dream that once seemed beyond reach. Whether I claim victory or not is beside the point; it's the proving ground for my perseverance, for my belief in second chances.

As the evening deepens, Cheryl sits silently by my side, her presence a comforting anchor. We don't need words; our shared history speaks volumes. At fourteen, I saw her and the world tilted. Her beauty wasn't just skin-deep—it radiated from within, lighting up the dreariest of rooms, igniting something fierce inside me. Her brothers, ever the sentinels, stood guard over their sister's heart. But fate has a way of bringing people together when the time is ripe, and eventually, it led me back to her, over thirty years later.

I steal a glance at Cheryl, the woman who saw me through the recovery from my darkest days. She draws a long breath from her cigarette, blowing smoke rings that drift skyward before dissipating. I think of those protective brothers of hers, now memories we honor, and I marvel at how life's tapestry unfolds—the patterns we never anticipate, the threads that lead us to where we're meant to be.

"Cheryl," I say softly, breaking the silence. "Do you remember the first time I tried to talk to you, and your brothers stepped in?"

She smiles, a knowing twinkle in her eyes. "How could I forget?" she replies, her voice tinged with nostalgia.

"Life's funny, isn't it? How it brings things full circle." I gaze back into the fire, its warmth seeping into my bones, chasing away the evening chill. "From high school crush to...well, everything we've built together."

"Everything we've faced so far," she adds with a squeeze of my hand.

"Everything we'll conquer," I promise with the quiet confidence of a man who knows he's no longer alone in his battles.

The stars peek through the velvet sky now, each one a testament to resilience—their light traveling vast distances, undeterred by the darkness. Like them, I've journeyed far from the brink of despair to a place of hope. And as the night wraps around us, I am content, filled with a sense of purpose and a belief in the infinite possibilities of tomorrow.

Watching the fire, I found my thoughts drifting to Cheryl's daughters—my stepdaughters—who had grown before our very eyes. They had transformed from wide-eyed teenagers into confident young women, each carving out their own slice of the world. I never had children of my own blood, but life, in its mysterious wisdom, had granted me the role of a stepfather and now a grandfather. The newest addition, a grandson with a cherubic face and a grip that already seemed to hold so many dreams, has given us fresh joy in our advancing years.

Time has etched its story onto Cheryl's face and mine; we have both felt the weight of years upon our shoulders. Yet as I look into her steady gaze, I see not just the traces of what has been but the promise of what is yet to come. We are sailing into the twilight of our lives, but we have each other, a sturdy vessel built on shared history and unwavering love.

There's a certain fortitude that comes with age, a resilience forged through decades of trials and triumphs. With every wrinkle, every silver strand of hair, we have accumulated not just years but wisdom—the kind that could only be earned, not taught. It was this wisdom we'd pass down to our beloved girls and their children, a legacy of lessons learned, and obstacles overcome.

"Life's a relentless teacher," I murmured, breaking the silence that had settled between us like a comforting blanket.

"Mmm," Cheryl agreed, a soft sigh escaping her lips as she extinguished her cigarette against the bench.

"Yet here we are," I continued, "still learning, still loving."

"Always," she whispered back, reaching for my hand, her touch as familiar as my own heartbeat.

As I gazed into the fire once more, I realized that hope, like the flames before us, needed fuel to keep burning bright. Our love, our family, our shared life—it was all kindling for the future, no matter how uncertain it may seem. And I knew, deep in the marrow of my bones, that together, we would endure whatever storms lay ahead, sheltering those we cherished with the strength of our combined spirits.

A smile crept across my face, warmth blooming in my chest, not just from the fire but from the realization of how lucky I truly was. Life had dealt me a remarkable hand, one I hadn't expected, pocket aces in the world of poker, but now couldn't imagine any other way. Resilience, hope, and a bit of luck—these had been my companions along the journey, and they would remain with me, guiding me through whatever chapters were left to write.

For all of this, I am eternally grateful. The words resonated within me, their truth as clear as the starry sky above. My life, once a tempest-tossed ship threatening to break upon jagged rocks, had found its harbor. I thank Jesus every day for taking the wheel, for steering me away from those perilous cliffs and into calmer waters.

I leaned back in my chair, feeling the reassuring presence of Cheryl beside me, her quiet breathing in sync with the tranquil night. How could I ever repay the blessings that had been showered upon me? A life more wonderful than I could have dreamed, graced by love, family, and a peace that once seemed unattainable.

Perhaps this book, these words spilling from my soul onto these pages, might serve as a lantern for others lost in their own darkness. It's my way of giving back, of showing that even when hope seems like a fragile, distant star, it's always there, waiting to be seized. By revealing my vulnerabilities, the mistakes and failures that are as much a part of me as my successes, maybe someone else will find the strength to persevere.

I pondered those who might stumble upon my story, who might see a glimmer of themselves in my struggles and triumphs. If you're one of those helped by this story, please let me know. My heart swells at the thought of connecting with another soul, of sharing the bond that struggle weaves between us all.

A gentle breeze stirs, carrying the scent of the damp earth and the lingering fragrance of summer blooms. And thank you so much for reading my story. The gratitude is profound, an echo of every heartbeat, every breath that I have been gifted since the day I chose to keep living.

I am truly honored and flattered that my story is one that is worth reading. The idea that my experiences, laid bare, might touch another life has filled me with a sense of purpose I have never known. And as I have said before, if it stops just one person, veteran or not, from taking their life, I will consider that to be the ultimate reward for my perseverance and faith.

The night deepened around us, the symphony of the evening lulling the world into a state of restful anticipation. Stars emerged, pinpricks of light in the vast canvas of the heavens, each one a silent witness to the countless stories unfolding below.

In the soft glow of the fire, with the love of my life by my side and the legacy of resilience woven into my being, I know that whatever lies ahead, hope will be my compass, luck my companion, and the shared strength of those I love my anchor. No matter the storms that might rage, together, we will navigate through them, emerging not just unscathed, but stronger for having faced them.

Resilience, hope, and a bit of luck—these were the threads of my life's tapestry, interwoven in a pattern uniquely mine, yet universally understood. They are the gifts I carry forth into each new day, the lessons I will pass on, and the legacy I will leave behind.

ABOUT THE AUTHOR

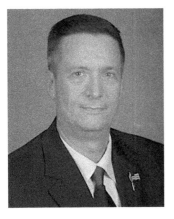

Robert, born in 1965, grew up poor in western Cleveland, Ohio, and then in Berea, Ohio. He has a unique background as he served in the army twice, from 1983 to 1992 and again at the age of forty-three, when the economy collapsed from 2008 to 2013. Following his first enlistment, he began a career in finance and banking, working various positions such as an insurance agent, branch manager, business banking officer, loan officer, and financial adviser.

Sadly, Robert was injured during his second enlistment and had to learn how to walk again. He was subsequently medically retired from the army. Despite this setback, Robert earned a degree in intelligence operations while on active duty with high honors. After retirement, he used the GI Bill to go back to college and graduated magna cum laude with a degree in business and criminal justice. He also obtained a certification in anti-money laundering.

In addition to his military and financial career, Robert has owned two businesses. The first was a financial planning firm that he started at the young age of twenty-three while also serving as the president of the Chamber of Commerce and board member of Rotary and Kiwanis clubs. His second business was a retail franchise that he purchased after retiring from the army.

After his second enlistment, Robert struggled with depression and anxiety and almost became one of the twenty-two veterans who tragically take their own lives every day. However, he has since found purpose and fulfillment in life. Currently retired for ten years, Robert has driven for Uber Black as a side job but spends most of his time playing Texas hold 'em poker tournaments online on ClubWPT and live locally—a passion that has led him to win some very large tournaments. He hopes to one day be considered a semiprofessional player and has recently joined the ClubWPT Stream Team and livestreams their tournaments once a week and as a backup.

Today, Robert's life is completely transformed from the dark place it once was when he nearly took his own life. He now shares his story in a book titled *Bobby, There Is Always Light at the End of the Tunnel* in hopes of preventing at least one suicide.

Printed in the USA
CPSIA information can be obtained
at www.ICGtesting.com
CBHW050628251124
17823CB00003B/8

9 798893 095494